CORE VALUES IN FAMILY MEDICINE

This new book explores the core values of family medicine nationally, regionally, and globally, to identify if and/or where there is consensus and where these diversify in relation to contextual factors. Aligned with the WHO's definition of primary healthcare and goal of universal health coverage and the United Nations Sustainable Development Goals, the book documents a global enquiry by teams of experts representing each world region on the vision, mission, core values and principles, and definition of family medicine in different countries. Each team has adopted different approaches and strategies in their exploration, findings, and conclusions.

A common identity for family doctors is important for research agendas, training, recognition of the specialty, and advocacy. However, there is much diversity within and across the regions in the training and the practice of the discipline of family medicine, reflected in the core values. The ultimate goal is a shared vocabulary of humanity for colleagues throughout the world, enriched rather than hindered by their differences.

The book will be an invaluable guide for general practitioners, family physicians, family medicine specialists, and other primary care doctors and a useful reference for other primary care health professionals including practice, school and other primary care nurses, medical assistants, paramedics, and community pharmacists. It will also serve as recommended or supplementary reading in undergraduate medical and nursing programmes, in university-based postgraduate courses and master programmes in relevant primary care–related topics, and in vocational training programmes in general practice/family medicine.

WONCA Family Medicine

About the series

The WONCA Family Medicine series is a collection of books written by worldwide experts and practitioners of family medicine, in collaboration with The World Organization of Family Doctors (WONCA). WONCA is a not-for-profit organization and was founded in 1972 by member organizations in 18 countries. It now has 118 Member Organizations in 131 countries and territories with membership of about 500,000 family doctors and more than 90 per cent of the world's population.

How To Do Primary Care Educational Research: A Practical Guide
Mehmet Akman, Valerie Wass, Felicity Goodyear-Smith

ICPC-3 International Classification of Primary Care: User Manual and Classification
Kees van Boven and Huib Ten Napel

Family Medicine in the Undergraduate Curriculum: Preparing Medical Students to Work in Evolving Health Care Systems
Valerie Wass, Victor Ng

Anxiety and Depression in Primary Care: International Perspectives
Sherina Mohd-Sidik, Felicity Goodyear-Smith

Core Values in Family Medicine: Inspiring Global Change
Anna Stavdal, Johann Agust Sigurdsson, Felicity Goodyear-Smith

Digital Health in Primary Care
Ana Luisa Neves, Liliana Laranjo

Challenges in Primary Mental Health Care
Christos Lionis, Christopher Dowrick

For more information about this series please visit: https://www.crcpress.com/WONCA-Family-Medicine/book-series/WONCA

CORE VALUES IN FAMILY MEDICINE

Inspiring Global Change

EDITED BY

Anna Stavdal, MD
University of Oslo, Oslo, Norway

Johann Agust Sigurdsson, MD, GP, Dr Med
University of Iceland, Reykjavik, Iceland, and Norwegian University
of Science and Technology (NTNU), Trondheim, Norway

Felicity Goodyear-Smith, MBChB, MGP, MD, FRNZCGP (Dist)
University of Auckland, Auckland, New Zealand

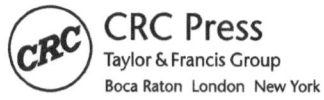

CRC Press
Taylor & Francis Group
Boca Raton London New York

CRC Press is an imprint of the
Taylor & Francis Group, an **informa** business

Designed cover image: Getty Images. Credit: BeholdingEye

First edition published 2026
by CRC Press
2385 NW Executive Center Drive, Suite 320, Boca Raton FL 33431

and by CRC Press
4 Park Square, Milton Park, Abingdon, Oxon, OX14 4RN

CRC Press is an imprint of Taylor & Francis Group, LLC

ISBN: **978-1-032-89333-4** (hbk)
ISBN: **978-1-032-89328-0** (pbk)
ISBN: **978-1-003-54235-3** (ebk)

DOI: 10.1201/9781003542353

Typeset in Minion Pro
by Apex CoVantage, LLC

Contents

Endorsement by the WONCA President

Core Values in Family Medicine: Inspiring Global Change presents an outcome from the World Organization of Family Doctors (WONCA) Global Core Values project. The project, launched in March 2023, has invited family doctors from around the world to reflect on their professional values, 'namely the values that mean most to them as a healthcare professional – both personally, within their specific context, and globally, within our shared profession'. Professional values serve to guide a discipline's members as a group, so this work is much needed by the discipline of family medicine.

Editors Anna Stavdal (Norway), Johann Agust Sigurdsson (Iceland), and Felicity Goodyear-Smith (New Zealand) have brought together a diverse range of 31 authors from all regions of the world to contribute their knowledge. In the book, each regional group describes their own unique approach to the task.

The differences in peoples, their cultures, and values across the world are reflected in the core values and principles in family medicine, as described in the various regional chapters. This diversity fosters a broader understanding and appreciation of various approaches to family medicine.

The editors conclude, 'We can be enriched rather than hampered by our differences. Within this heterogeneity, we need a common identity for the recognition of our specialty and for advocacy, a common language of our humanity enabling us to connect with our colleagues across the world'.

Dr Monty Kent-Hughes, WONCA's first president from 1972, said that 'the future of our professional discipline will depend on our ability to work together in the service of humanity.'

The establishment of our shared identity though the Global Core Values project will contribute greatly to our ability to work together and achieve a high impact on global health. I recommend this book to all family doctor colleagues wanting to understand the professional values of our discipline in their own country and region, as well as to better understand colleagues from other parts of the world.

Associate Professor Karen M. Flegg
Australian National University
Rural Clinical School
World Organization of Family Doctors
(WONCA) World President

Foreword

The concept of the family physician emerged in the mid-20th century as a response to the increasing specialization within medicine, which had led to a decline in the number of general practitioners and a fragmentation of patient care. This shift prompted concerns about the erosion of the patient–doctor relationship and the need for comprehensive, continuous care.

The idea of a family doctor has steadily evolved, gaining recognition and clarity. This progression has refined not only the global understanding of the vital role family doctors play in healthcare systems but also the core qualities and competencies that define the profession. Family physicians have come to be recognized as essential providers of comprehensive, patient-centred care, bridging gaps between different medical disciplines and ensuring continuity of care across all stages of life.

The World Organization of Family Doctors (WONCA) has been the global engine powering the genesis of the fine-tuned specialty. We must, however, admit that the growth of the specialty has not been at the same pace across all regions of the world. Sections of Europe, Australia, and the Americas have had a more rapid evolution compared with Asia and Africa.

Discussions and collaborative planning efforts focused on vision, missions, core values, and the definition of family medicine in contemporary contexts have taken place across various countries and regions over the past few decades. I have always been deeply passionate about core values of family physicians and have personally authored a published paper on the subject.

The Global Core Values project delves into the fundamental principles that define primary care and family medicine. It examines a wide range of interconnected concepts, acknowledging that interpretations and definitions may vary across different contexts and healthcare systems.

By identifying and analyzing these core principles, the Global Core Values project helps healthcare professionals, policymakers, and educators align their practices with universally recognized ideals, fostering consistency in care delivery. Additionally, recognizing variations in interpretation allows for adaptability across diverse healthcare settings, ensuring that these values remain relevant and applicable in different cultural, social, and systemic contexts.

This collaborative project acknowledges the invaluable contributions of leading experts in family medicine, whose dedication and expertise have played a pivotal role in shaping the development of a groundbreaking new specialty. The book covers all seven regions of WONCA – Africa, Asia Pacific, South Asia, East Mediterranean, Europe, North America, and South America.

It is my distinct honour to acknowledge the efforts of the esteemed leaders of this project – Dr Anna Stavdal, Immediate Past President of WONCA; Professor Felicity Goodyear-Smith, the longest-serving Chair of WONCA's Research Working Party; and their colleague, Johann Sigurdsson, Emeritus Professor from the University of Iceland. Their dedicated leadership, along with a team of global family doctors, was instrumental in the successful completion of this project.

This book will guide the development of curricula, standardization of training methods, and creation of benchmarks for global standards of practice for the specialty. It will be invaluable in informing policymakers, healthcare leaders, and various institutions about the significance of family physicians in strengthening primary healthcare and improving public health outcomes. For practising family physicians, this book serves as a reaffirmation of their professional identity, inspiring commitment to their core mission and encouraging lifelong learning. It educates patients, communities, and stakeholders on the essential role family doctors play in promoting holistic healthcare, prevention, and long-term patient well-being. Finally, scholars and researchers in primary care can use the book as a foundation for further studies on the evolution, impact, and future directions of family medicine.

Professor Henry J. O. Lawson
Head of Family Medicine Unit,
University of Ghana Medical School, Accra, Ghana
Vice Rector, Ghana College of Physicians and Surgeons
Past President, WONCA Africa Region (2016–18)

Acknowledgements

Many thanks to all who contributed to our project and to this book, including all members of regional teams who are not authors and the participants of the conference workshops and surveys. Our gratitude to the WONCA secretariat, especially Andrea Zard, for answering tricky questions and giving updated information.

A special thanks to the guest speakers at our online meetings: Kay Mohanna, the professor of values-based healthcare education at Three Counties Medical School, UK, and Kurt C. Stange, a distinguished university professor at the Department of Family Medicine and Community Health, School of Medicine, Case Western Reserve University, USA, for their words of wisdom and their generosity of time, giving their talks twice across different time zones.

The editors

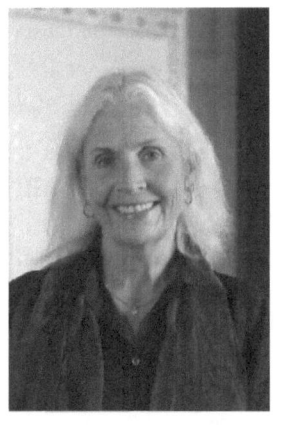

Anna Stavdal, MD, is a family doctor based in Oslo, Norway, where she has been providing care to patients since 1989. In addition to her clinical practice, she holds the position of Associate Professor at Oslo University, where she actively contributes to the education and training of future healthcare professionals. With primary areas of interest in health systems and the core values of family medicine, she is a passionate advocate for family medicine and primary care, and she actively engages in public debates, sharing her expertise through columns and speaking engagements.

Anna Stavdal is Honorary Fellow of the College of General Practice in Sri Lanka and holds an honorary doctorate at the University of Oslo, Finland. Her leadership roles within family medicine organizations since 1994 demonstrate her commitment to advancing the field on various levels. She has held influential positions in Norwegian, Nordic, European, and global family medicine organizations. She assumed the prestigious position of President of the World Organization of Family Doctors (WONCA) from November 2021. Since November 2023 she holds the office of Past President. Her role as the head of this global organization underscores her ability to shape and guide initiatives that promote family medicine worldwide.

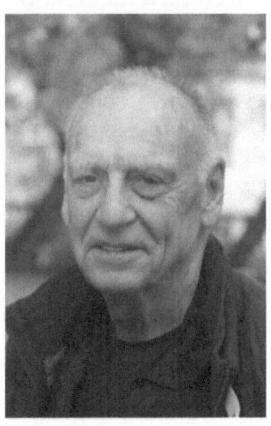

Johann Agust Sigurdsson, MD, GP, Dr Med, has worked as a general practitioner for 40 years. Now emeritus, he served as a professor of family medicine at the University of Iceland in Reykjavik for 23 years and as a professor in general practice at the Norwegian University of Science and Technology (NTNU), Trondheim, Norway, for 5 years. His primary research areas include cardiovascular epidemiology, infectious diseases, antimicrobial resistance, modelling studies on the implementation of clinical guidelines, childbirth and health, ethical issues and dilemmas, and multimorbidity.

Throughout his career, Johann has been actively involved in the professional development of general practice/family medicine (GP/FM) in the Nordic countries. He was the National Editor of the *Scandinavian Journal of Primary Health Care* during 1986–2010, president of three Nordic congresses on general practice, and played a key role in implementing specialist training in general practice in Iceland. Additionally, he served as Chair of the Nordic Federation of General Practice from 2017 to 2023. During this time, the Nordic colleges, alongside Anna Stavdal, President of WONCA Europe and later WONCA World, took the lead in advancing the moral intent and core values of GP/FM among the Nordic colleges and in WONCA Europe.

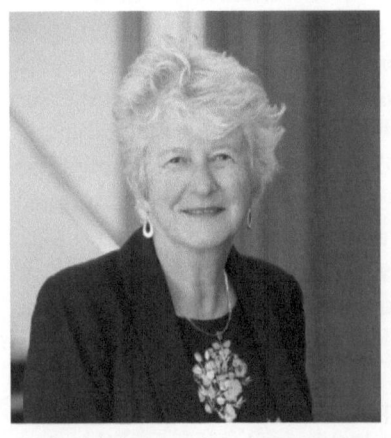

Felicity Goodyear-Smith, MBChB, MGP, MD, FRNZCGP (Dist), is a general practitioner and professor of general practice and primary healthcare at the University of Auckland, Auckland, New Zealand. She has a long involvement with WONCA including past Chair of its Working Party on Research. She has previously co-edited five books in the WONCA Family Medicine series and has also contributed chapters to three other books in this series. Dr Goodyear-Smith was the founding editor-in-chief of the *Journal of Primary Health Care*, which she has been co-editing since 2022. She has published over 350 peer-reviewed papers as well as a number of books and book chapters.

She has always seen that a core feature of family medicine is the trusted relationship between clinician and patient and family, as well as with other members of the primary care team. She was excited to become a member of the steering group for this Global Core Values project, which extends the previous enquiry on the nature of our discipline from Nordic and European countries to all regions of the world. It is a privilege to work with colleagues across the globe. While this book is one result, more important is the ongoing process of engagement.

Contributors

Faisal A. AlNaser, MBBS, FPC, MICGP, FRCGP, FFPH, FAM (USA), PhD
President Bahrain Family Medicine Association, Honorary Professor of Family Medicine
Department of Primary Care and Public Health, Imperial College, London
Juffair, Bahrain

Zainab Mohammad Anjarwala, MBBS, FCPS, MRCGP (Int)
Assistant Professor
Department of Family Medicine
Dow University of Health Sciences
Karachi, Pakistan

Helen Alter, MD
Family Physician
Järveotsa Perearstikeskus
Tallinn, Estonia

Nana Kwame Ayisi-Boateng, MBChB, MPhil, FGCP
Senior Lecturer and Family Medicine Consultant
University Hospital
Kwame Nkrumah University of Science and Technology
Kumasi, Ghana

Innocent K. Besigye, MBChB, MMed
Regional lead for Africa, Senior Lecturer, and Family Physician
Department of Family Medicine
Makerere University
Kampala, Uganda

Rodney Destine, MD
Family Physician and Consultant, President of Haitian Association of Family Physicians
Saint-Marc, Haiti

Otto Hamann Echeverri, MD
Specialist in Family Medicine
Dean, and Professor
Fundación Universitaria Juan N Corpas
Bogotá, Colombia

Catherine Gathu, MBChB, MMed, MSc, FHEA
Assistant Professor and Consultant Family Physician
Department of Family Medicine
Medical College, East Africa
Aga Khan University
Nairobi, Kenya

María Belén Giménez, MD
Professor and Family Medicine
    Specialist
Service of Family Medicine
    Universidad Nacional de
    Asunción
Asunción, Paraguay

**Felicity Goodyear-Smith, MBChB,
MGP, MD, FRNZCGP (Dist)**
Professor and General Practitioner
    Department of General Practice
    and Primary Health Care,
    University of Auckland
Auckland, New Zealand

Nena Kopcavar Gucek, MD, PhD
Assistant Professor, General
    Practitioner/Family Physician
Department of Family Medicine
    Medical Faculty, University
    of Ljubljana and Community
    Medical Center
Jubljana, Slovenia

Fabiano Gonçalves Guimarães, MD
President of the Brazilian Society
    of Family and Community
    Medicine
Rio de Janeiro, Brazil

**Pramendra Prasad Gupta, MBBS,
MD (General Practice and
Emergency Medicine)**
Additional Professor
    BP Koirala Institute of Health
    Sciences
Dharan, Nepal

**Nagwa Nashat Hegazy, MSc, MD,
DHPE, FAIMER**
Professor of Family Medicine
    Family Medicine Department
    Menoufia University
    Menoufia, Egypt

Paula Henry, MBBS, MPH, MBA
Family Physician
    Family Medicine Doctors' Inn
    Port of Spain, Trinidad and Tobago

Machiko Inoue, MD, MPH, PhD
Vice President of Japan
    Primary Care Association
    Professor, and Family
    Physician
Department of Family and
    Community Medicine
Hamamatsu University School of
    Medicine
Hamamatsu, Japan

Mónica Álvarez Jaramillo, MD
Family Medicine and Health
    Management Specialist and
    Associate Professor
Fundación Universitaria Juan N
    Corpas
Bogotá, Colombia

**Raman Kumar, MBBS, DNB
(Family Medicine)**
Director
    Institute of Family Medicine and
    Primary Care, Greater Noida
    West
Uttar Pradesh, India

Johanna Lynch, MBBS, Grad Cert (Grief & Loss), PhD, FRACGP, FASPM
Senior Lecturer and Family Doctor
General Practice Clinical Unit
Medical School
The University of Queensland
Brisbane, Queensland, Australia

Nina Monteiro, MD
General Practitioner/Family Physician
USF Bom Porto, ULS Santo António
Porto, Portugal

Keneilwe Motlhatlhedi, MBChB, MMed
Lecturer
Department of Family Medicine
and Public Health
University of Botswana
Gaborone, Botswana

Leilanie Nicodemus, MD
Professor
Department of Family and
Community Medicine
College of Medicine University of
the Philippines
Manila, Philippines

Sairat Noknoy, MD, MSc Public Health (Health Services Research), FRCFPT
Regional Lead for Asia Pacific, Vice
President of Royal College of
Family Physicians of Thailand
Bangkok, Thailand

Mona Osman, MD, MPH, MBA, MHPE, DipIBLM
Regional Lead for East
Mediterranean, President
Lebanese Society of Family
Medicine, Assistant Professor of
Family Medicine
Department of Family Medicine
American University of
Beirut
Beirut, Lebanon

David Ponka, MD CM, CCFP (EM), FCFP, MSc
Professor, Assistant Dean, Global
Health
Faculty of Medicine, University
of Ottawa
Ottawa, Canada

Jacqueline Ponzo, MD, MSc
Family and Community Medicine
Specialist
Regional Lead for
Iberoamericana-CIMF and
Added Professor
Academic Unit of Family
and Community Medicine
Universidad de la República
Montevideo, Uruguay

Sankha Randenikumara, MBBS, MCGP
Regional Lead for South Asia and
Chief Family Physician
The Family Health Clinic
Colombo, Sri Lanka

Katharina Schmalstieg-Bahr, MD
General Practitioner and Researcher
Department of General Practice
and Primary Care
University Medical Center
Hamburg-Eppendorf
Hamburg, Germany

Wadeia Sharief, MD
Professor of Family Medicine,
President of Emirates Family
Medicine Society
Director Medical Education and
Research Department in Dubai
Health Authority
Dubai, United Arab Emirates

**Johann Agust Sigurdsson, MD, GP,
Dr Med**
Emeritus Professor in Family
Medicine and Family Physician
University of Iceland
Reykjavik, Iceland

Anna Stavdal, MD
Past President of WONCA
Associate Professor, and Family
Medicine Specialist
Department of General Practice
University of Oslo
Oslo, Norway

Harry H.X. Wang, MD, PhD
Professor of Public Health
School of Public Health
Sun Yat-sen University
Guangzhou, China

Kim Yu, MD, FAAFP, DABFM
PRIME National Strategy
Consultant
American Board of Family
Medicine
Lexington, Kentucky

Dorien Zwart, MD, PhD
Regional Lead for Europe, General
Practitioner/Family Physician
Professor of General Practice/
Family Medicine
Department of General
Practice & Nursing Sciences
Julius Center for Health
Sciences and Primary Care
University Medical Center
Utrecht University
Utrecht, The Netherlands

CHAPTER 1

Introduction to the Core Values project

Anna Stavdal, Johann Agust Sigurdsson, and Felicity Goodyear-Smith

AIM OF THE GLOBAL CORE VALUES PROJECT

Brainstorming processes on vision, missions, core values, and the definition of family medicine in contemporary contexts have been conducted in different countries and regions in the past few decades, including in Norway, the Nordic countries, and subsequently Europe, as outlined in the following chapter. Drawing on this existing work, this project involves a global brainstorming process and actions taken on core values and the definition of the specialty of family medicine.

A common identity for family doctors is important for research agendas, training, recognition of the specialty, and advocacy. However, there is much diversity within and across the regions in the training and the practice of our discipline, which may be reflected in our core values. This book documents the different approaches and strategies adopted by each region in their exploration, findings, and conclusions. The ultimate goal is a shared vocabulary of our humanity, enabling us to reach out to colleagues throughout the world, enriched rather than hindered by our differences.

THE NATURE OF PRIMARY HEALTHCARE, PRIMARY CARE, AND FAMILY MEDICINE/GENERAL PRACTICE

While the terms are often used interchangeably, primary care (PC) needs to be distinguished from primary healthcare (PHC). The World Health

DOI: 10.1201/9781003542353-1

Organization (WHO) defines PHC as an approach to health policy and service provision that includes both individual-based care and population-level public health and policy.[1] Population health includes health promotion, disease prevention, public health, and rehabilitation services. PHC also incorporates wide multi-sectorial functions including public health measures and community-based social services.[2] PC services sit with PHC. PC involves first contact with people and their families in their pursuit of healthcare and health. Individual care encompasses the health and wellbeing of the whole person and their family throughout all ages and stages of life.[3]

Family doctors, in some countries known as general practitioners, are uniquely vocationally trained among medical disciplines to serve as first-contact practitioners and leaders of a PC team. Family doctors are taught to address multiple medical and social issues for the same patient and to integrate care for the individual and family across the broadest span of PHC. Family doctors may also rely on the other health professionals in their PC team (including nurses, midwives, pharmacists, mental health workers, and many others), dependent on setting and context. Strong communication lines between, and close collaboration with, different PC professionals in the team increase the effectiveness of PC.[4]

Complaints and conditions may not have precise diagnoses. In 1982 Gayle Stephens described how complaints and conditions which:

- Are obscure, vague, undifferentiated.
- Arise from life-threatening disease.
- Seem out of proportion to physical or lab findings.
- Are unusual, bizarre, non-physiologic, non-anatomical.
- Are persistent and disabling.
- Are associated with marked anxiety or mood change.
- Arise from life change, conflict, or stress.
- Might require risky and therapeutic procedures.
- Arise from conditions which may be managed electively.
- Are incurable.
- Involve habits and lifestyle of the patient.
- Require moral or ethical decisions.

all require the unique managerial skills of a wise and compassionate family doctor, beyond standard operating procedures or a cookbook approach to diagnosis and therapy.[5]

In his Williams Pickles lecture in 1996, Ian McWhinney explained the ways family medicine and other PC disciplines differ from other medical specialties:

1. Family medicine is the only medical discipline to define itself in terms of relationships, especially the doctor–patient relationship (PC is relational rather than transactional).
2. Family doctors tend to think in terms of individual patients rather than generalised abstractions (patient rather than disease focused).
3. Family medicine is based on an organismic rather than a mechanistic metaphor of biology and disease (mechanistic is linear – a cause for each disease, whereas organismic is non-linear with multiple feedback loops between organism and environment and between all levels of the organism; causal networks which maintain an illness and inhibit healing may be different from the causes which initiated it, and these may include the organism's own maladaptive behaviour).
4. Family practice is the only major field which transcends the dualistic division between mind and body.[6]

PC involves managing patients' health needs, their undifferentiated complaints, concerns, and issues in the context of their lives. Generalism has been defined as the:

> professional philosophy of healthcare practice, described as 'expertise in whole person medicine'. The 'expertise' of generalism relates to an approach to care which is person not disease oriented; taking a continuous rather than an episodic view; integrating biomedical and biographical understanding of illness; to support decisions which recognise health as a resource for living and not an end in itself.[7]

Building on international consensus that described generalism as expertise in whole-person care that integrates both biology and biography,[7] Lynch and colleagues describe the craft of generalism as having whole-person scope, relational process, and pragmatic healing goals that require integrative wisdom.[8] Reductionist approaches that focus on single diseases ignore the multi-faceted causality of illness in the face of complexity such as multi-morbidity, persistent physical symptoms, and social determinants of health.

It is important that PC is integrated within the health system. The WHO defined health as 'a state of complete physical, mental and social well-being and not merely the absence of disease or infirmity' in 1948.[9] This definition was reaffirmed by the Alma Ata Declaration of 1978.[10] The 2018 Astana Declaration at the Global Conference on Primary Health Care organized by the WHO and UNICEF acknowledged the Alma Ata Declaration, which made a strong commitment to the fundamental role of strong PHC for population health.[11] The Astana Declaration presented three interconnected components:

1. Empowering populations and communities that can prioritise and co-design responses to their health needs.
2. High-quality PC, integrated with public health.
3. Multi-sectoral policy and action.

Integrated health systems with PC as a core function are required for its implementation, which must be linked to community services.[3] Patient-centred care requires an integrated approach to the patient's health journey within the health system from primary to secondary and tertiary care and back as well as to community agencies and social care. This requires quality communications via referral and discharge letters and documentation of dialogue and cooperation.

Key principles of primary care

In the 1970s Barara Starfield specified four unique key principles which differentiate PC from secondary care: first contact, comprehensiveness, coordination, and longitudinality (continuity) of care,[12] known as the '4Cs'. She demonstrated that these functions lead to better health outcomes, lower costs, and greater equity in health.[13,14] PC should serve as the main entry point and interface between the population and the health system, the users' preferential contact, and the main entrance to the healthcare system.[15] The family doctor works as the hub between hospitals, community health, and social care and public health services. Ideally, continuity of care is the patient's experience of a 'continuous caring relationship' with an identified healthcare professional. When a patient is known to their family doctor, there is increased patient safety and quality of care over time. While continuity of provider is not always possible, a patient-centred PC team can also provide continuity of care. The family doctor is the only member of the team trained to take the full responsibility of the patient's primary medical care, whereas the other members of the PC team are trained in specific elements of the patient's overall care.

Comprehensiveness of care can be considered along different dimensions:

1. The scope or range of services offered and available (promotion, prevention, early diagnosis, curative, rehabilitative, and palliative).
2. The spectrum of population needs that can be addressed along the life course, which includes the ability of practitioners to care for patients at any stage of their lives ('cradle to grave') and in any care setting.
3. The holistic approach to care, including psychosocial needs.

4. The depth of services (severity or complexity of illness managed) and breadth (acute and chronic) of conditions managed by the PC team.
5. The navigation of the health system which reduces the risk of fragmented care.[16]

Coordination of care consists of leading, organizing, and integrating patient care across different locations, specialties, and phases of care. The family doctor integrates vertical disease-oriented approaches with longitudinal, horizontal provision of healthcare tailored to the individual patient in the context of their lives.[15]

More recently, Starfield's core functions of PC have been expanded with the additional three 'Cs' of patient-centredness, community engagement, and complexity.[17]

Patient-centredness

The structuring principle of PC is patient-centredness. Patient-centred care focuses on the individual patient's particular healthcare needs, with the goal to empower patients to become active participants in their care.[18] The key tasks of the clinician in a patient-centred consultation are to establish rapport, elicit the patient's agenda (reasons for the visit), decide with the patient the priority in addressing the issues (acknowledging that some may need to wait until a later time), undertake as required the clinical process of eliciting symptoms and targeted examination to formulate differential diagnoses and exclude serious conditions that require acute action, arrive at an agreed plan with the patient through the active process of share decision-making, and finally discuss follow-up arrangements. The emphasis is on a partnership between the clinician and the patient, and their family where appropriate, to ensure that decisions respect their wants, needs, and preferences.

The patient's agenda may not be the presenting issue. This may be the most socially acceptable explanation for coming, but the main reason for the visit may be introduced at the end of the consultation or go unvoiced and may be the most vague or embarrassing. The PC provider's agenda is to address the patient's health concerns within the time constraints of the consultation. Family doctors may start the consultation with open-ended questions such as 'How can I help you today?', 'What do you need from me today?', and 'What brought you here today?' to elicit the patient's primary concern. Where the patient has more issues than can be addressed in a single consultation, these can be prioritized so that the most important items are dealt with on this occasion.[19]

In patient-centred care, clinicians engage professionally with their patients' current life situations, biographical stories, beliefs, worries, and hopes.[20] This helps to recognize the links between social factors and sickness and to deepen understanding of how life and life events leave their imprint on the human body. To safeguard their long-term resilience as caregivers, providers also attend to their own wellbeing.

Shared decision-making

For patients to make informed decisions on their investigation or treatment preferences, PC providers need to give them clinically relevant information, communicated in a way that they can understand and make sense of.[21] Patients' questions are:

1. What will happen to me (what is the natural history of my condition)?
2. What are my choices? What will happen if we do nothing, just wait and watch?
3. What are the possible benefits and harms of these different choices?
4. How likely are each of those benefits and harms to happen to me?

For the health provider, shared decision-making is central to patient-centred care:

1. It helps patients have greater understanding of options, realistic expectations, and to make choices aligned with their own values and preferences.
2. It is important to communicate benefits and risks in ways patients can understand.
3. Communication should take patients' health literacy, preferences, and circumstances into account.
4. The question is 'What shall we decide?'
5. Note that shared decision-making will not always be possible, and in some circumstances, patients may want their clinicians to make decisions for them.

People-centred and person-centred care

There has been a shift in the use of terms from patient-centred to person-centred and people-centred care, although as yet there are no precise definitions to differentiate these. Person-centred care is said to consider a person's needs, values, and preferences and identifies that the healthcare professional and person must work together to plan optimal care.[22]

People-centred care is a broader principle than patient-centred care. WHO defines it as care that is focused and organized around the health needs and expectations of people and communities rather than on diseases.[23] It extends from the individual patient to families, communities, and society – everyone in the continuum of care. It includes attention to the health of people in their communities and their crucial role in shaping health policy and health services. All should have an equal voice. The rationale is that patients should not be reduced to, nor defined by, their disease, illness, or condition. They are people with individual preferences, needs, and abilities who are full partners in their care. They are persons, not cases.[24]

KEY CONCEPTS

The Global Core Values project explores the core values of primary care and family medicine. It covers many overlapping concepts, and again, there may be variations in definition. We present our understanding of various terms and concepts for the benefit of this project, acknowledging that these may not be definitive definitions.

Values and principles

Values are a set of ethical beliefs and preferences that determine the sense of right and wrong and serve as a guide for human behaviour. They are basic convictions of what individuals or social groups consider right, good, or desirable.[25] Values are not specific to given objects or situations – they are stable and enduring beliefs that generally require prolonged social or educational processes to change.[26] In contrast, attitudes and beliefs vary with different situations and usually refer to evaluation of specific objects, actions, or situations with some degree of favour or disfavour.

Values can be personal (held individually), collective (held by a group), or institutional (held by an organization). Having values means that you hold yourself to account and maintain a certain level of professionalism and care in all that you do. They can be considered qualities to strive for.

Principles are built upon values and are the rules or beliefs that govern behaviour – the response or action in which to express values. If the value is honesty, a principle might be to never tell lies. Principles are specific to a particular field and provide a framework for how to act in certain situations. In the context of family medicine, the principle of patient-centredness requires the core value of compassion to make the human connection. Specific skills include establishing rapport, eliciting the patient agenda, prioritizing, clinical care, and shared decision-making. This is embedded in the principles of comprehensiveness, continuity, and coordination.

Professional values serve to guide a discipline's members as a group. They shape the discipline's principles, identity, and beliefs and lie behind professional codes, explaining and justifying the specific duties that professionals bear. 'Statements of values indicate what is important; statements of professional or organisational standards define what to consider as good or acceptable.'[27] However, while healthcare is a value-laden activity, opinions may differ on what 'doing the right thing' is. There may be conflicting views about whose best interest, or in multidisciplinary teams, there may be a diversity of profession-specific values.[28]

Purpose, vision, and mission

The purpose, vision, and mission of an organization are the why, what, and how of its existence. The purpose of an organization is why it exists, its goal or objectives. Organizations such as family medicine professional bodies often have vision and mission statements. The vision is what the organization and its members are aiming for, the big picture of what they hope to achieve in line with their goal. The mission is how the organization functions – what it does, whom it serves, and what it needs to do to accomplish its vision. Advocacy is one means to achieve vision at an organizational level. At the individual member level, reflective practice can be a means to achieve vision. Core values can determine behaviour during the process.

Skills, competencies, and attributes

Skills can be defined as strengths or proficiencies gained through training and experience. In the context of family medicine and PC, communication, clinical, and management skills are core.

The principal core skill for PC is communication – between family doctor and patient and between family doctor and other health providers. Trust is a cornerstone of the patient–family doctor relationship with indisputable benefits. Trust must be earned over time through continuity of care. Family doctors get to know patients as people, their life situation, stories, beliefs, worries, and hopes. This helps use the best evidence and recognize the links between social factors and sickness and to deepen understanding of how life and life events are inscribed in the human body.

Key communication skills are:

1. Early identification of the patient's main problem (the problem is not necessarily the same as the disease).
2. Putting other problems in a priority order and formulating a plan for their longer-term assessment and management.
3. Formulating a strategy for dealing with the problem in the time available.
4. Focusing on the decisions which have to be taken at this visit.
5. Selecting the most efficient strategy for arriving at these decisions, including how to ensure shared decision-making.[6]

In many health systems, family doctors have a gatekeeping role, regulating patients' access to secondary health services. While gatekeeping is frequently viewed as a strategy to reduce health service use and health expenditure, it can also serve as a useful function of preventing unnecessary investigations and over-treatment. A key competency for family doctors is to know when to refer a patient for a specialist consultation.

In regard to clinical skills, family medicine uses a generalist problem-based rather than disease-based approach to eliciting symptoms, examining for signs and requesting investigations. History-taking and physical examination are tailored to the patient's presentation and to prior knowledge of their health and social history. Presentations may be undifferentiated with vague symptoms and diagnostic uncertainty. The focus may be on diagnosis of exclusion (ruling out serious conditions) rather than reaching a definitive diagnosis. The role of time and 'watchful waiting' reduces over-treatment – reassess to see whether symptoms resolve or worsen or new ones appear. Too many tests can cause harm, especially among healthy people who might be defined as sick or given a diagnosis that does not benefit their health. Over-testing can lead to unfair distribution of health services, as it steals resources from the sick.

Management skills are also important. The consultation is managed to ensure the patient's agenda is revealed; issues are prioritized; the clinical process of assessment, diagnosis, explanation, and negotiation is followed; and the consultation concludes with an agreed plan of action and follow-up. There needs to be a systematic approach to clinical record-keeping, with appropriate investigations requested and referral letters written, and results and replies are reviewed, actioned, and filed in a timely manner.

Competencies can be defined as sets of demonstrable proficiencies and abilities to achieve a goal. They typically combine skills, abilities, and knowledge and can include the specific behaviours needed to complete a task. Attributes can be defined as characteristics. After decades of discussion (within Leeuwenhorst, the European Academy of Teachers in General Practice [EURACT] and others), WONCA Europe published their first version of 'The European Definition of General Practice' in 2002.[29] It defined the key features of the discipline of general practice, the role of the general practitioner, and described the core competencies of the general practitioner/family physician. In 2004 the Swiss College of Primary Care developed the WONCA Tree as a graphic representation of general family practice which depicts the relationship between six core competencies (branches) and 12 attributes (leaves). The Tree was incorporated into the European definition statement and has since been revised by WONCA Europe in 2011 and 2023. The latest revision of the European Definition was published in 2024.[30]

WORLD ORGANIZATION OF FAMILY DOCTORS (WONCA)

The acronym WONCA comes from the first five initials of the World Organization of National Colleges, Academies and Academic Associations of General Practitioners/Family Physicians, shortened to the World Organization of Family Doctors.

WONCA's mission is 'to improve the quality of life of the peoples of the world through defining and promoting its values, including respect for universal human rights and including gender equity, and by fostering high standards of care in general practice/family medicine by:

- Promoting personal, comprehensive and continuing care for the individual and the family in the context of the community and society.
- Promoting equity through the equitable treatment, inclusion and meaningful advancement of all groups of people, particularly women and girls, in the context of all healthcare and other societal initiatives.
- Encouraging and supporting the development of academic organizations of general practitioners/family physicians.
- Providing a forum for exchange of knowledge and information between Member Organizations and between general practitioners/family physicians.
- Representing the policies and the educational, research and service provision activities of general practitioners/family physicians to other world organizations and forums concerned with health and medical care.'

WONCA was founded in 1972 by member organizations (such as colleges of family medicine) in 18 countries. There are now 133 member organizations from 111 countries and territories. WONCA is organized into seven world regions (Africa, Asia Pacific, East Mediterranean, Europe, Iberoamericana-CIMF, North America, and South Asia), each of which has their own regional council and runs their own regional activities, including conferences.

REFERENCES

1. World Health Organization. Chapter 7: Health systems: Principled integrated care. World Health Report 2003 Shaping the Future. Geneva, Switzerland: WHO, 2003.
2. Muldoon LK, Hogg WE, Levitt M. Primary Care (PC) and Primary Health Care (PHC): What is the difference? *Can J Public Health* 2006;97(5):409–11.
3. Olde Hartman TC, Bazemore A, Etz R, et al. Developing measures to capture the true value of primary care. *BJGP Open* 2021;5(2). https://doi.org/10.3399/bjgpo.2020.0152
4. Sixty-Second World Health Assembly. Primary health care, including health system strengthening. WHA6212. Geneva, Switzerland: WHO, 2009:3.
5. Stephens G. The Intellectual Basis of Family Practice. Tucson, AZ, USA: Winter Publishing Company Inc. 1982.
6. McWhinney IR. William pickles lecture 1996: The importance of being different. *Br J Gen Pract* 1996;46(408):433–6.
7. Reeve J, Dowrick CF, Freeman GK, et al. Examining the practice of generalist expertise: A qualitative study identifying constraints and solutions. *JRSM Short Rep* 2013;4(12):2042533313510155. https://doi.org/10.1177/2042533313510155

8. Lynch JM, van Driel M, Meredith P, et al. The craft of generalism: clinical skills and attitudes for whole person care. *J Eval Clin Pract* 2022;28(6):1187–94. https://doi.org/10.1111/jep.13624

9. World Health Organization. WHO Constitution. Geneva, 1948.

10. World Health Organization. Declaration of Alma-Ata: International Conference on Primary Health Care. Alma-Ata, USSR: WHO, 1978.

11. World Health Organization. Declaration of Astana: From Alma-Ata towards Universal Health Coverage and the Sustainable Development Goals. Astana, Kazakhstan: Global Conference on Primary Health Care, 2018:12.

12. Starfield B. Measuring the uniqueness of primary care. *J Ambulatory Care Manage* 1979;2(3):91–9.

13. Starfield B, Shi L. Policy relevant determinants of health: An international perspective. *Health Policy* 2002;60(3):201–18.

14. Starfield B. Primary care and health: A cross-national comparison. *JAMA* 1991;266(16):2268–71.

15. Jimenez G, Matchar D, Koh GCH, et al. Revisiting the four core functions (4Cs) of primary care: Operational definitions and complexities. *Prim Health Care Res Dev* 2021;22:e68. https://doi.org/10.1017/S1463423621000669

16. Macinko J, Starfield B, Shi L. Quantifying the health benefits of primary care physician supply in the United States. *Int J Health Serv* 2007;37(1):111–26. https://doi.org/10.2190/3431-G6T7-37M8-P224

17. Bazemore A, Grunert T. Sailing the 7C's: Starfield revisited as a foundation of family medicine residency redesign. *Fam Med* 2021;53(7):506–15. https://doi.org/10.22454/FamMed.2021.383659

18. Levenstein JH, McCracken EC, McWhinney IR, et al. The patient-centred clinical method. 1. A model for the doctor-patient interaction in family medicine. *Fam Pract* 1986;3(1):24–30. https://doi.org/10.1093/fampra/3.1.24

19. Sathanapally H, Sidhu M, Fahami R, et al. Priorities of patients with multimorbidity and of clinicians regarding treatment and health outcomes: A systematic mixed studies review. *BMJ Open* 2020;10(2):e033445. https://doi.org/10.1136/bmjopen-2019-033445

20. Silverman J, Kurtz S, Draper J. Skills for Communicating with Patients. 3rd ed. London: CRC Press 2013:328.

21. Krist AH, Tong ST, Aycock RA, et al. Engaging patients in decision-making and behavior change to promote prevention. *Stud Health Technol Inform* 2017;240:284–302.

22. Barnett N. Person-centred over patient-centred care: Not just semantics. *Clinical Pharmacist* 2018;10. https://doi.org/10.1211/CP.2018.20204578

23. World Health Organization. People-Centred Health Care: A Policy Framework. Geneva: WHO, 2007:28.

24. Health Standards Organization. Patient- vs People-Centred Care: What's the Difference? Ottawa, Canada: HSO 2020 [updated 12 Jan. Available from: https://healthstandards.org/general-updates/people-vs-patient-centred-care-whats-difference/ accessed Aug 2024]

25. Rokeach M. The Nature of Human Values. New York: Free Press 1973.

26. Bergman MM. A theoretical note on the differences between attitudes, opinions, and values. *Swiss Polit Sci Rev* 1998;4(2):81–93. https://doi.org/10.1002/j.1662-6370.1998.tb00239.x

27. Sigurdsson JA, Beich A, Stavdal A. Our core values will endure. *Scand J Prim Health Care* 2020;38(4):363–6. https://doi.org/10.1080/02813432.2020.1842676

28. Mohanna K. Values based practice: A framework for thinking with. *Educ Prim Care* 2017;28(4):192–6. https://doi.org/10.1080/14739879.2017.1313689

29. WONCA Europe. The European Definition of General Practice/Family Medicine, 2002:35.
30. Windak A, Rochfort A, Jacquet J. The revised European definition of general practice/family medicine: A pivotal role of one health, planetary health and sustainable development goals. *Eur J Gen Pract* 2024;30(1):2306936. https://doi.org/10.1080/138147 88.2024.2306936

CHAPTER 2

Processes of exploration into the core values of family medicine

Anna Stavdal, Johann Agust Sigurdsson, and Felicity Goodyear-Smith

DEVELOPMENT OF THE DISCIPLINE

General practice as a discipline has a relatively short history compared with other medical specialities. The term 'general practitioner' was first used in 1809 and was soon in common use.[1] Although Professor Thomson of the Westminster Medical Society argued against medical specialization when he wrote in 1828, 'The general practitioner [should] be looked upon as at the head of the profession',[2] most British medical practitioners were members of the Royal Colleges of Physicians or Surgeons or of the Society of Apothecaries.[3] Until the mid-20th century, physicians and surgeons specialized and held hospital appointments, from which community-based doctors were mostly excluded.[4]

The College of General Practitioners was founded in Britain in 1952, soon followed by a number of others, including the College of General Practice of Canada in 1954, the Dutch College of General Practitioners in 1956, the Australian College of General Practitioners in 1958, the Philippine Academy of Family Medicine in 1960, the Danish College of General Practice in 1970, and the College of General Practitioners Singapore in 1971. The World Organization of Family Doctors (WONCA) was founded in 1972 with member organizations in 18 countries. Many more countries subsequently established family medicine professional colleges and/

DOI: 10.1201/9781003542353-2

or training programmes, for example, Malaysia and Sweden in 1973, New Zealand in 1974, Iceland and Spain in 1978, Sri Lanka in 1979, and Norway and Finland in 1983. In Latin America, postgraduate training programmes in family medicine were started in Mexico, Panama, and Bolivia in the 1970s.[5]

Initially these doctors were called general practitioners (GPs), but later some countries, such as the United States and Canada, called community-based doctors who had not undergone any postgraduate training GPs, reserving the term 'family physician' for those who have completed a family medicine training programme. Often confusion related to terminology (such as GP, family or primary care or community doctor) causes challenges in policy dialogues. Due to traditions and culture, it has proved hard to agree on one term for the physician who is trained in accordance with the basic principles outlined in Chapter 1.

Traditionally, general practice was not a discipline taught to undergraduate medical students. The first Chair in General Practice was established in Edinburgh, Scotland, in 1963, and it took nine more years before an English Chair in General Practice was founded in Manchester in 1972. During the 1960s, universities in the Netherlands (University of Utrecht), Canada (Western University, Ontario), and Norway (University of Oslo) followed with their own university general practice departments and academic professors.[6] Since then, the academic standing of the discipline has grown, with departments of general practice and primary healthcare in many universities across the globe, involved in undergraduate medical and postgraduate training programmes, as well as in doctoral programmes and active engagement in research.

By 2024, 133 colleges and academies of family medicine (member organizations) in 111 countries and territories belonged to WONCA. As can be seen in Figure 2.1, there is uneven distribution of high-income countries. Lower-income countries, where strong primary care is likely to contribute most to better health outcomes for all, are found disproportionately in Africa, South Asia, and South America. Countries without family medicine training programmes (coloured grey) are predominantly in Africa.

Many of the general practice/family medicine colleges developed vision and mission statements, definitions of family medicine and core professional competencies, and values and principles. However, there were widely diverging definitions within the different languages, with distinctive cultural implications not necessarily shared between countries.[7]

One of the explicit objectives for WONCA is that undergraduate and postgraduate training in family medicine is established in every medical faculty in the world.

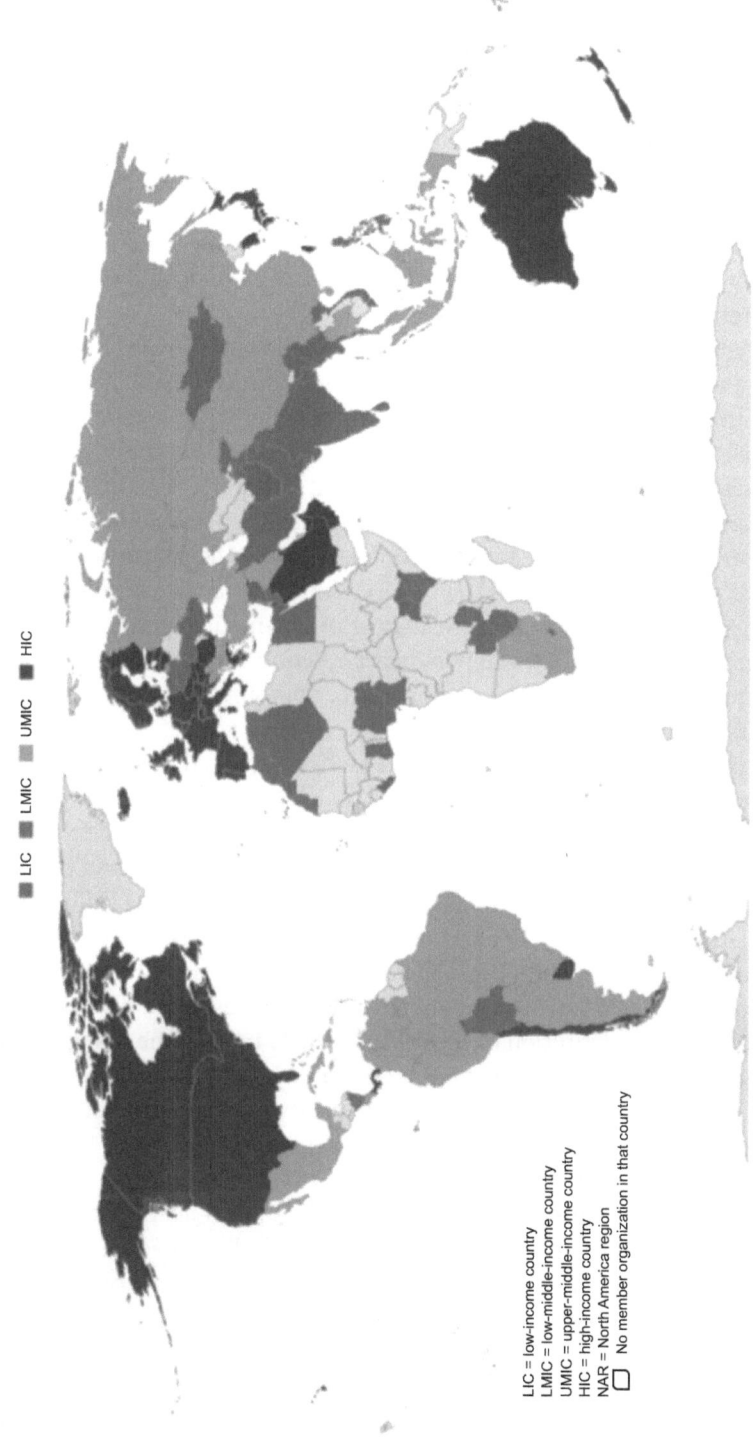

LIC = low-income country
LMIC = low-middle-income country
UMIC = upper-middle-income country
HIC = high-income country
NAR = North America region
☐ No member organization in that country

FIGURE 2.1 Distribution of World Bank income level ranking of the 111 WONCA member countries.

EARLY NATIONAL AND REGIONAL EXPLORATIONS INTO DEFINITIONS AND VALUES OF GENERAL PRACTICE

The first GP organization, the International Society of General Practice (Societas Internationalis Medicinae Generalis or SIMG), was founded in 1959 in Vienna. Originally for individual members, many national colleges and societies which shared the aims of SIMG subsequently became corporate members. SIMG was an academic organization which aimed to raise the international standard of patient care and academic standing of general practice by focusing on the scientific and medical background of the emerging discipline.[8]

In the 1970s through to the 1990s the Royal College of General Practitioners (RCGP) and the Dutch College of General Practitioners (DCGP/NHG) led the way in Europe in developing the philosophy of general practice/family medicine. The RCGP published the book *The Future General Practitioner: Learning and Teaching* in 1972. This could be considered visionary, centring more than ever before on the importance of the GP in the healthcare system, with a focus on the patient as a person seen in a context.[9] In 1975 Richardson argued in the *British Medical Journal (BMJ)* that general practice has a philosophy of medical care distinguishable from that of other medical specialities, being 'the doctor of first contact, the personal and continuing responsibility, and the comprehensive nature of general practice combines to create a balance of values and judgments'.[10]

Also in 1972 the European General Practice Research Workshop was set up, stimulated by a conference in 1971 for countries bordering on the North Sea. Belgium, Denmark, Finland, France, West Germany, the Netherlands, Norway, Sweden, and the UK were the first member countries, and the group started to explore shared meanings of terminology.[11] In 1974 the DCGP/NHG, in association with the RCGP and the Danish College, ran a conference in the Netherlands which led to the establishment of the Leeuwenhorst European Study group. Twelve European countries were represented, and the group developed a shared definition of the role of the GP. In 1982 the first group was dissolved, and the New Leeuwenhorst Group expanded to include members from 22 European countries, focused primarily on teaching and learning. Later on the group was renamed the European Academy of Teachers in General Practice (EURACT).

In 1981 Ian McWhinney, the family physician and academic known as Canada's 'Founding Father of Family Medicine', described the principles of family medicine as 'a distinctive worldview – a system of values and an approach to problems that is identifiably different from that of other disciplines'.[12]

The RCGP set up a Working Party looking at the role of the GP in the context of illness and disease in relation to environment and psychosocial aspects. This culminated in their 1985 report *What Sort of Doctor?*[13] The Working Party agreed upon nine value statements:

1. The doctor tries to render a personal service, which is comprehensive and continuing.
2. In his practice arrangements he balances his own convenience against that of his patients, takes into account his responsibility to the wider practice community, and is mindful of the interests of society at large.
3. He accepts the obligation to maintain his own mental and physical health.
4. He puts a high value on communication skills.
5. He subjects his work to critical self-scrutiny and peer review and accepts a commitment to improve his skills and widen his range of services in response to newly disclosed needs.
6. He recognizes that researching his discipline and teaching others are part of his professional obligations.
7. He sees that part of his professional role is to bring about a measure of independence: he encourages self-help and keeps in bounds his own need to be needed.
8. His clinical decisions reflect the true long-term interests of his patients.
9. He is careful to preserve confidentiality.

The authors explain that 'for convenience, "he" is used to denote "he or she" throughout'.

At a meeting in Portugal in 1994, members of WONCA and SIMG decided to merge their organizations into the European Society of General Practice/Family Medicine. WONCA Europe was inaugurated in 1995 in Strasbourg, France, and included the three European network organizations existing at that time: EURACT, the European General Practice Research Workshop (EGPRW), and the European Working Party on Quality in Family Practice (EQuiP).

In a 2002 editorial in the *BMJ*, Pendleton and King argued for the importance of medical organizations to explicitly declare their values[14]:

> Values are deeply held views that act as guiding principles for individuals and organisations. When they are declared and followed they are the basis of trust. When they are left unstated they are inferred from observable behaviour. When they are stated and not followed trust is broken.

SPECIFIC INVESTIGATIONS INTO THE CORE VALUES AND PRINCIPLES OF GENERAL PRACTICE

In 2001, after considerable discussion and meetings with members, the Norwegian College of General Practice (NSAM), led by Dr Anna Stavdal, produced a poster listing the core values and principles for general practice as seven theses (*Sju teser*) published in Norwegian. The seven theses translated roughly as:

1. Maintain the doctor–patient relationship.
2. Do what is most important, prioritizing patients with conditions in need of treatment and sparing patients from wrongfully being treated as sick.
3. Give the most to those most in need.
4. Use words that promote health in the individual.
5. Participate in continuing education, research, and professional development.
6. Describe your experiences from practice.
7. Take the lead.

Inspired by the Norwegian College declaration of their core values, the Danish College of General Practice (DSAM), under the leadership of Dr Anders Beich, engaged in a large-scale 'vision process' involving hundreds of GPs. This resulted in the *Pejlemærker for faget almen medicin* (*Guidelines for the Field of General Medicine*) published in Danish in 2016, which contained seven similar statements to those from Norway.[15]

In 2005 a collaboration of family medicine institutions in Norway, Denmark, Sweden, Iceland, and Finland had been formalised by the establishment of the Nordic Federation of General Practice (NFGP).[16] In 2017, the NFGP decided to reexamine their vision and mission statements, formulate their core values and guiding principles, and attempt to merge the Norwegian *Sju teser* and the Danish *Pejlemærker for faget almen medicin* into an English-language statement on which they could all agree.[7] Hundreds of Nordic GPs participated in workshops and digital exchanges, with a diversity of opinions and suggestions emerging that was enriching and greatly appreciated.[15] In 2020, the English rendering of the Nordic GPs' shared understanding was agreed, and the Nordic statement 'Core Values and Principles of Nordic Family Medicine' was produced. The poster listed seven core values and principles[17]:

1. We promote continuity of doctor–patient relationships as a central organising principle.
2. We provide timely diagnosis and avoid unnecessary tests and overtreatment. Disease prevention and health promotion are integrated into our daily activities.
3. We prioritise those whose needs for healthcare are greatest.
4. We practice person-centred medicine, emphasising dialogue, context, and the best evidence available.

5. We remain committed to education, research, and quality development.
6. We recognise that social strain, deprivation, and traumatic experiences increase people's susceptibility to disease, and we speak out on relevant issues.
7. We collaborate across professions and disciplines while also taking care not to blur the lines of responsibility.

A further explanation is provided to the right of each item. A video on the core values of general practice was also produced for the YouTube platform (https://www.youtube.com/watch?v=cbwtk3Ax0E4). In 2021, versions of these Nordic core values were reproduced in Icelandic, Swedish, and Finnish.

The core values in family medicine in the context of several lower-income countries were also explored. A study of Ukrainian family doctors using a Delphi panel process found six core values emerged from the process: comprehensive approach, care coordination, first recourse, continuity of care, integrated approach, and patient- and family-centred care.[18] A purposive sample of African family medicine practitioners in academia, public service, private practice, and clinical training across Central, East, North, South, and West Africa were also recruited into a study using the Delphi technique.[19] The final five core values from this process were identiifed as comprehensive care, continuity of care, collaborative care, patient-centred care, and lifelong learning, with similarities to those determined by the Nordic countries and Ulkraine.

The DCGP/NHG published their *Position Paper: Core Values of General Practice/Family Medicine* in 2011, with a revision in 2019. Focusing on the discipline in 2011, the college wrote:

> General practice medicine is generalist, patient-oriented, continuous care. These core values are inextricably linked to each other. The quality of general practice/family medicine can only be described by viewing these core values in the mutual connection. The GPs actions at the practice are based on these core values.[20]

In 2022, WONCA Europe developed a further process with a working group and workshops. After much deliberation, WONCA Europe adopted core values and principles as a framework of reference for the region adapted from the Nordic one.[21] This acknowledged that general practice/family medicine may be practised in different contexts according to the characteristics of each health system, country, or community. Figure 2.2 shows the Norwegian, Danish, Nordic, and European posters.

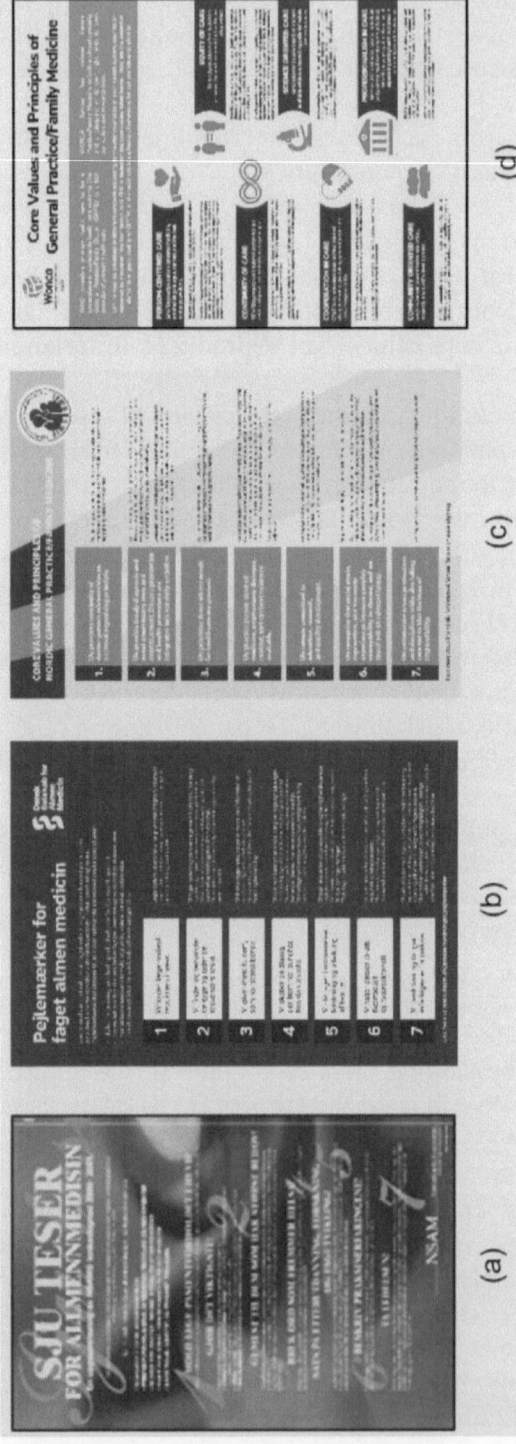

FIGURE 2.2 Core value posters. (a) *Sju teser*, (b) *Pejlemærker for faget almen medicin*, (c) Nordic core values, and (d) European core values.

THE GLOBAL CORE VALUES PROJECT: INSPIRING GLOBAL CHANGE

In March 2023, Anna Stavdal launched the WONCA Global Core Values project in her president's message in the WONCA newsletter. She said that 'for a definition of family medicine to impact identity, members need to have a stake in it, that sense of ownership that comes from having won it for themselves.' A designated email address was included for members to respond to with the invitation: 'Please reflect on the values that mean most to you as a healthcare professional – both personally, within your specific context, and globally, within our shared profession'.

An initial exercise was carried out by Prof Felicity Goodyear-Smith in June/July 2023 to explore existing statements of vision, mission, definition of family medicine, and core values and principles of all WONCA member organizations by going through accessible online resources. Organizations were entered into an Excel spreadsheet and the relevant data extracted from their websites or available organization documents. Figure 2.3 shows the seven WONCA regions of the world. Countries in grey are those without member organizations.

Organizations were scored as to whether they had nothing recorded/available (0); the mission and vision of the organization but not the discipline (1); further mission, vision, and description but not comprehensive (2); or a full mission, vision, and description of family medicine, core values and principles (3). Where there was more than one member organization in a country, the one with the most comprehensive coverage was selected. No information was available for 38% of organizations, 32% had organizational information only, 13% had more detail, and just over a quarter, 26%, provided full information. Figure 2.4 shows the global distribution of these records.

A steering group was established, composed of Anna Stavdal; Johann Agust Sigurdsson, an emeritus professor of family medicine, University of Iceland; and Felicity Goodyear-Smith, professor of general practice and primary healthcare at the University of Auckland, New Zealand.

The next step was the appointment of regional leaders for Africa, Asia Pacific, East Mediterranean, Europe, North America, South America/Ibero-Americana, and South Asia to further explore the core values and principles of the member organizations and family doctors in the countries in their respective regions. Key members of the WONCA Working Party on Research who were approached showed considerable enthusiasm to take part in this project.

All leads were asked to recruit members to their team from other countries in their region, looking for diversity with respect to country income level and other cultural aspects as much as possible, as well as personal characteristics such as age, gender, rural versus urban, and academic versus clinical practice backgrounds. Each lead is responsible for subsequent chapters in this book, outlining their processes and findings for their respective regions.

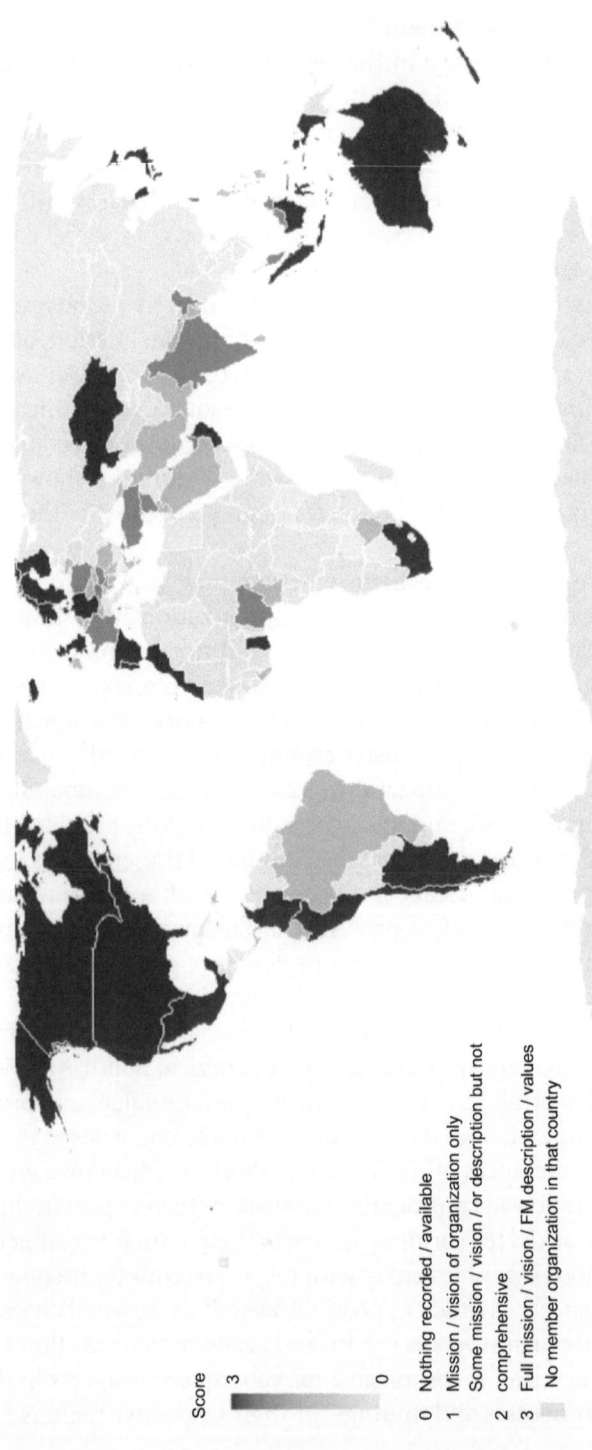

Score

3

0

0 Nothing recorded / available
1 Mission / vision of organization only
2 Some mission / vision / or description but not comprehensive
3 Full mission / vision / FM description / values
   No member organization in that country

FIGURE 2.3 WONCA regions of the world.

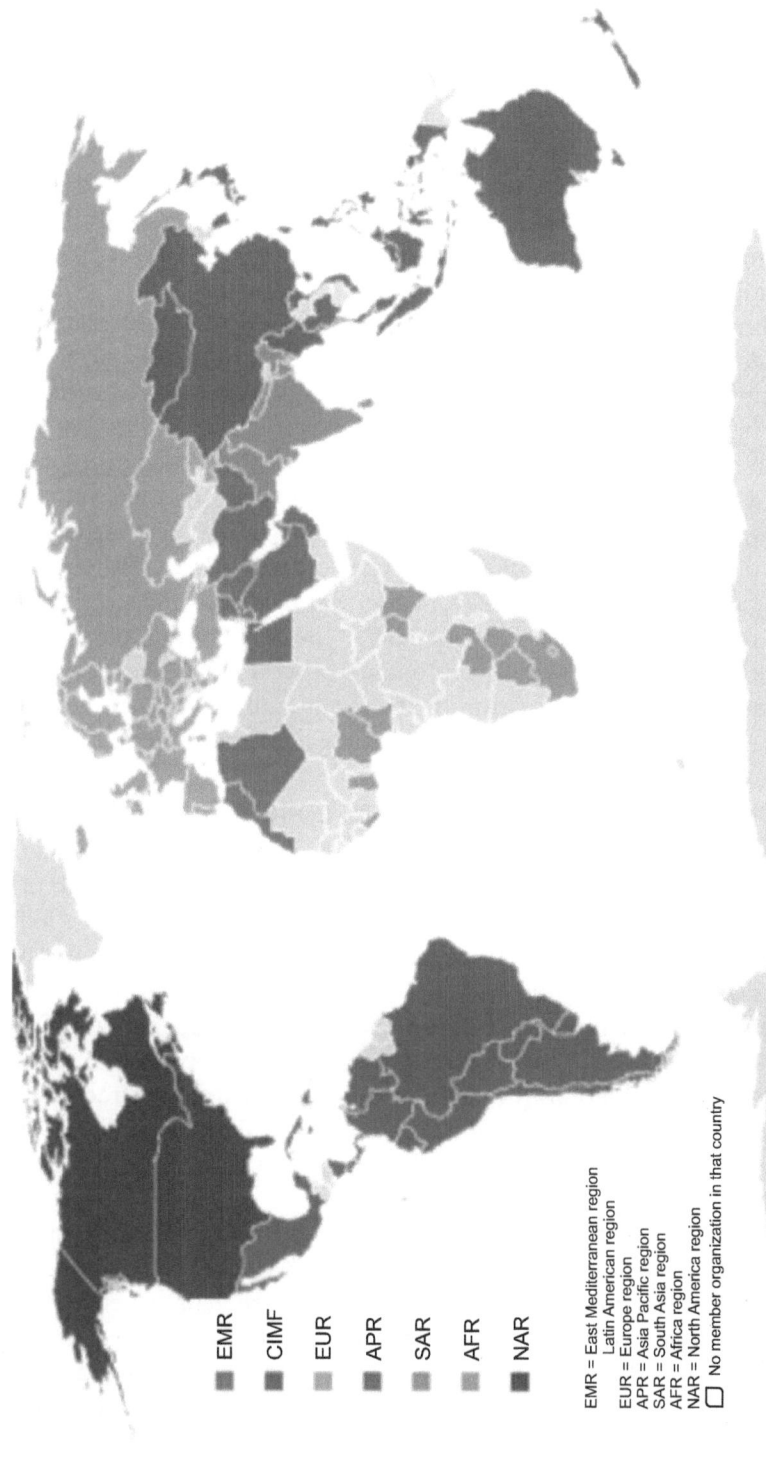

EMR = East Mediterranean region
      Latin American region
EUR = Europe region
APR = Asia Pacific region
SAR = South Asia region
AFR = Africa region
NAR = North America region
☐ No member organization in that country

FIGURE 2.4 Member organization record of mission, vision, core values, and description of family medicine.

Regular global group meetings conducted on the Zoom platform then commenced. Throughout the project, these were run twice at 12 hours apart at times to suit either participants in Asia or the Americas but also at sociable-enough times (morning and evening) for steering committee members in Europe and New Zealand to attend both meetings. Recordings were made and disseminated for those who could not make either meeting to review. Leaders and their teams were all invited, and if a lead was unavailable for either time slot, they were asked to delegate a team member to provide an update for their region.

The final establishment and launch of the global project took place at the WONCA World Conference in Sydney, Australia, in October 2024. In her keynote presentation, President Anna Stavdal called for a shared vocabulary needed in uncertain times. She argued that a broadening of the core values in family medicine and a values-based action plan are needed to respond to the many challenges facing family doctors: geopolitical stress, environmental disasters, healthcare workforce shortages, commercialisation of medical care, and the digitisation and dehumanising of person-centred care. Following this address, an augural face-to-face workshop was held with the steering committee, regional leads, and team members. The background, purpose, and timeline were outlined, along the proposed process for the next two years, culminating with a final session of the group and their outcomes at the WONCA World Conference in Lisbon, Portugal, in September 2025.

ONGOING PROCESSES OF THE GLOBAL CORE VALUES PROJECT IN 2024 AND 2025

A proposal was prepared for the project to form the basis of a book in the WONCA Family Medicine Series published by Taylor & Francis, and following its submission and peer review, the proposal was accepted and this book contract was secured in June 2024.

Core value workshops by the teams have been conducted at WONCA regional meetings. Each region developed their own approach to the task, including communication with member organizations, data extraction from documentations, and surveys of member organizations or family doctors. Details of the regional workshops and processes are outlined in the succeeding chapters.

Regular online meetings took place, with comprehensive regional updates. Along with the current WONCA president, Karen Flegg, the president elect, Viviana Martinez-Bianchi, and Nina Monteiro, liaison person for the WONCA Lisbon Conference 2025, joined the group as *ex officio* members.

Each region had their own approach to the task, which included running workshops at the WONCA regional conferences. Their processes are outlined in the following regional chapters. To help promote further discussion and deeper exploration, the steering committee invited selected experts as guest speakers to talk about professional values by providing an external independent view to broaden thinking.

REFERENCES

1. Loudon I. Medical Care and the General Practitioner 1750–1850. Oxford: Clarendon Press 1986:354.
2. Thomson A. Westminster medical society. *Lancet* 1828;11(271):176–7.
3. Goodyear-Smith F. History of primary care research. In: Goodyear-Smith F, Mash B, eds. International Perspectives on Primary Care Research. London, England: Routledge 2016.
4. Tait I. History of the College. London: Royal College of General Practitioners, 2002.
5. World Health Organization, World Organization of Family Doctors. Making medical practice and education more relevant to people's needs: The contribution of the family doctor. Ontario, Canada: Joint WHO-WONCA Conference, 1994:103.
6. Straand J, Wit N. The transition of general practice into an academic discipline: Tracing the origins through the first four professors in general practice/family medicine. *Scand J Prim Health Care* 2024;42(3):483–92. https://doi.org/10.1080/0281 3432.2024.2335537
7. Sigurdsson JA, Beich A, Stavdal A. A saga-in-progress: Challenges and milestones on our way toward the Nordic core values and principles of family medicine/general practice. *Front Med* 2021;8:681612. https://doi.org/10.3389/fmed.2021.681612
8. Meyer R. From SIMG to WONCA Europe – ESGP/FM. *Prim Care* 2009;9(15):268.
9. Royal College of General Practitioners. The Future General Practitioner – Learning and Teaching. London: BMJ 1972.
10. Richardson IM. The value of a university department of general practice. *BMJ* 1975;4(5999):740–2. https://doi.org/10.1136/bmj.4.5999.740
11. Horder J. The RCGP and other countries: A beginning. *Br J Gen Pract* 1990;40(334):206–9.
12. McWhinney I. A Textbook of Family Medicine. Oxford, UK: Oxford University Press 1989.
13. What Sort of Doctor? Working Party. What Sort of Doctor? Report from General Practice. London: RCGP 1985:23.
14. Pendleton D, King J. Values and leadership. *Br Med J* 2002;325(7376):1352–5. https://doi.org/10.1136/bmj.325.7376.1352
15. Sigurdsson JA, Beich A, Stavdal A. Our core values will endure. *Scand J Prim Health Care* 2020;38(4):363–6. https://doi.org/10.1080/02813432.2020.1842676
16. Stavdal A. The Nordic federation of general practice. *Scand J Prim Health Care* 2005;23(3):129. https://doi.org/10.1080/02813430500217106
17. Nordic Federation of General Practice (NFGP). Core values and principles of Nordic general practice/family medicine. *Scand J Prim Health Care* 2020;38(4):367–8. https://doi.org/10.1080/02813432.2020.1842674
18. Kolesnyk P, Bayen S, Shushman I, et al. Identification and ranking of core values in family medicine: A mixed methods study from Ukraine. *Front Med* 2021;8. https://doi.org/10.3389/fmed.2021.646276
19. Lawson HJO, Nortey DNN. Core values of family physicians and general practitioners in the African context. *Front Med* 2021;8. https://doi.org/10.3389/fmed.2021.667144
20. van der Horst HE, de Wit N. Redefining the core values and tasks of GPs in the Netherlands. *Br J Gen Pract* 2020;70(690):38–9. https://doi.org/10.3399/bjgp20X707681
21. WONCA Europe. The European Definition of General Practice/Family Medicine, 2002:35.

CHAPTER 3

Family medicine core values in Africa

Innocent K. Besigye,
Keneilwe Motlhatlhedi,
Catherine Gathu,
and Nana Kwame Ayisi-Boateng

REGIONAL DESCRIPTION

The WONCA Africa region (WAR) covers sub-Saharan Africa (SSA) and consists of three major regions of the continent: Western Africa, Eastern Africa, and Southern Africa. SSA is composed of 48 countries (Figure 3.1): 23 low-income countries, 18 lower-middle-income countries, 6 upper-middle-income countries, and 1 high-income country (the island state of Seychelles) per the 2024 World Bank classification. Among these countries, there are only 15 WONCA member organizations in 12 countries, with Nigeria having 3 member organizations and all others having 1.

Geographically, Sudan, Djibouti, Eritrea, and Somalia are located in SSA. Different organizations include different countries in the regions of Africa and the East Mediterranean – there is no standardized definition. Historically the World Health Organization (WHO) has classified Sudan, Djibouti, and Somalia in their East Mediterranean Regional Office (EMRO), but Eritrea in their African region. In 2011, following a civil war, Sudan was divided into the Republic of Sudan (Sudan) and South Sudan. Initially, both countries remained classified in the EMRO, but South Sudan requested to be reassigned to the African region. This request was accepted, and South Sudan is now part of the WHO African region.

DOI: 10.1201/9781003542353-3

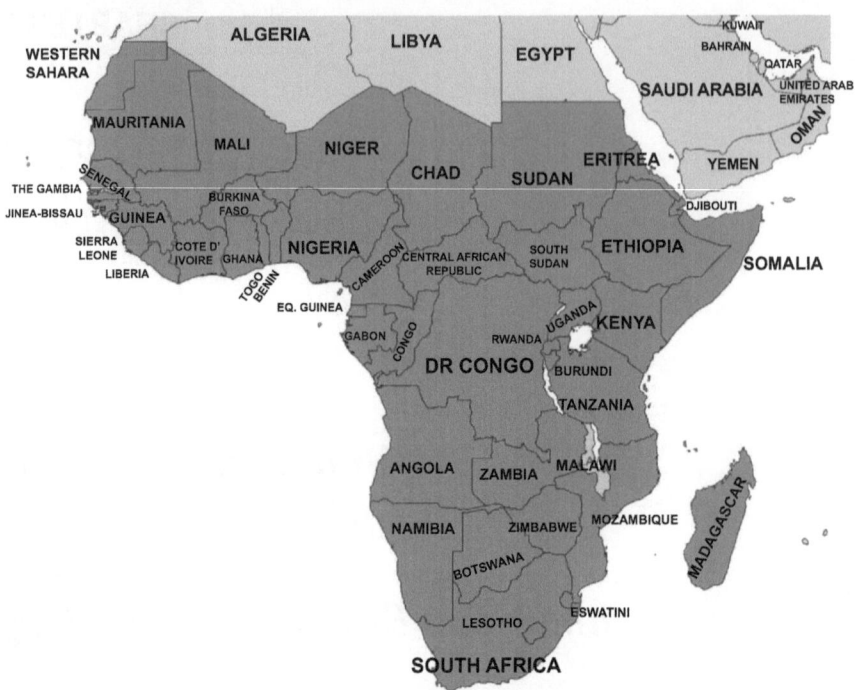

FIGURE 3.1 Map of Africa showing sub-Saharan African countries.

Source: mapchart.net

Because geographically the Republic of Sudan (Sudan), South Sudan, Djibouti, Eritrea, and Somalia are located in SSA, we include them as countries in our African region. None of these countries have member organizations in WONCA. However, WONCA EMR has always been aligned with the WHO EMRO, so note that Sudan, South Sudan, Djibouti, and Somalia are also included in their chapter.

Apart from Ethiopia, all other countries in SSA are former colonies of European countries. Despite the end of colonialism more than 50 years ago, its effects still exist, with significant influence on culture, geopolitical, and socioeconomic situations. As a result, there are several official languages spoken among the countries, mainly English, French, and Portuguese. The colonial history contributes to differences in lifestyle, norms, and beliefs. Such differences make it difficult to create cohesion among countries. For example, there is disproportionate lower inclusion of Francophone- and Portuguese-speaking countries within the WONCA Africa family.

Family medicine is relatively new in most SSA countries. Family medicine training started in the 1960s in South Africa and in the 1970s in Nigeria.[1,2]

In other countries, family medicine training started in the 1990s, albeit slowly, with the training in some countries and some institutions stopping altogether.[3] Currently, there is rapid growth of the discipline, evidenced by many countries commencing the training and inclusion of family medicine within their undergraduate curricula.[3,4] This rapid growth is likely to accelerate exponentially with the establishment of the Eastern Central and Southern Africa College of Family Physicians.[5]

As the discipline evolves, there is need for a clear definition for better understanding among different stakeholders. This is because family medicine is highly contextual with no one model working across different settings. However, the values and principles are likely to be the same. Definition of family medicine, its values, and principles in Africa has been part of the conversation since the early 2000s.[6,7]

ACCESS TO FAMILY PHYSICIANS

Access to family physicians in SSA is limited due to low numbers. In most countries, the total number of family physicians on the specialist register is fewer than 100. Table 3.1 shows the number of registered family physicians per member country and other related access parameters.

In most cases, family physicians in SSA are not first-contact clinicians. They are mainly working in district hospitals providing general medical care, including obstetrics and surgical emergencies. First-contact primary care is mainly provided by nurses, mid-level clinicians (clinical officers/associates), and non-postgraduate trained generalists known as medical officers. The primary healthcare (PHC) teams are poorly developed, and primary care lacks efficient gatekeeping. This makes primary care fragmented and uncoordinated, lacking comprehensiveness, continuity, and person-centredness. The family physicians working in such circumstances have to exhibit flexibility and adaptation to the circumstances but still keep the values and principles of the discipline.

PROCESSES

The Africa region team was composed of representatives from Western, Eastern, and Southern Africa. The team members regularly met online to discuss the methods and strategies of data collection. Online information by member organizations was collected where available. The data collected focused on the vision, mission, and goals of family medicine in a country. Member organizations where no such information was found online were contacted directly to provide relevant information that might inform understanding of family medicine core values. A workshop was held at the eighth WAR conference in Nairobi, Kenya, to ascertain the views of the participants

TABLE 3.1 Country Population Characteristic and Number of Registered Family Physicians

Country	Income Range	Population (millions)	Population Density (per km²)	Urbanization (%)	Number of Registered FPs
Angola	Lower middle income	37	30	68	14
Botswana	Upper middle income	2.4	4.4	72	40
Cameroon	Lower middle income	28.4	60.9	59	16
DRC	Low income	106	46.6	47	60
Eswatini	Lower middle income	1.2	70.9	25	6
Ethiopia	Low income	126	132	23	55
Gambia	Low income	2.7	273	64	6
Ghana	Lower middle income	33	148.9	59	365
Kenya	Lower middle income	55	99.2	29	59
Lesotho	Lower middle income	2.3	77	30.4	14
Liberia	Low income	5.4	58	53.6	23
Malawi	Low income	21	230	18.3	40
Mozambique	Low income	34	44	39	15
Namibia	Upper middle income	3.03	4	53.7	4
Nigeria	Lower middle income	227	250	54	1,200
Sierra Leone	Low income	8.5	117	44	7
Somaliland	Low income	6.2	29	-	29
South Africa	Upper middle income	68	53	68.8	1,064
Tanzania	Lower middle income	66.6	75	37	10
Uganda	Low income	46	243	26	50
Zambia	Lower middle income	20	27	46	15
Zimbabwe	Lower middle income	16.3	43	32	3

Key: FP = family physician.

Source: Online sources as of 2024, with some country verbal communication for number of registered family physicians.

on the subject, as well as their understanding of family medicine from their respective contexts. The collected information was collated and analyzed thematically to discern the contemporary core values of family medicine within the African context. A literature review was also conducted to explore what has already been described for the region.

FINDINGS

Family medicine core values have been part of the conversation in Africa for decades now. The founding fathers of family medicine in Africa were equally concerned at that time and argued that there was a need to define family medicine in the African context.[6-8] Initial family medicine models in Africa were Eurocentric, based on American and European approaches to primary care. Current trends show that there have been progressive efforts to reorient family medicine training and practice towards the African context. Following are the family medicine core values described for the African region.

Principle of continuity of care

In most African countries, primary care is not well developed, with most health systems fragmented, focused on vertical programmes in secondary and tertiary care, and lacking gatekeeping. Family physicians working in these health systems drawing on global evidence on the contribution of continuity of care to better health outcomes strive to promote it. They put emphasis on establishing a trusted relationship with their patients as a key ingredient to continuity of care. In some settings, they share their telephone contacts with their patients for easy personal reach when necessary. Relational continuity is difficult in the public health sector, as practitioners are occasionally transferred or rotate from one facility to another. Informational continuity is mostly through health facility or patient-held handwritten records, with little or no access to an electronic health record system.

Principle of coordination of care

African family physicians acknowledge that they cannot address and manage all the health needs of every individual. Some people in populations they serve will need to be referred for diagnostic and/or therapeutic purposes. In some cases, the family physician arranges with the specialist or the facility where the person is being referred to ensure an easy reception. However, the family physicians retain the responsibility of coordinating the care team and follow-up. In some cases, the family doctor remains available to the patient for guidance where necessary. This strengthens the doctor–patient relationship.

Principle of comprehensive care

In many African countries, human resources for health are way below the WHO recommendations.[9] Team-based healthcare is limited. Therefore, family physicians in some instances are working solo and struggle to meet the diverse needs of individuals, families, and communities. African family physicians strive to have broad knowledge and extended procedural skills to provide the needed comprehensive care. The level of the required comprehensiveness provided by the family physician depends on where one is practising. Family physicians practising in rural and remote areas have more requirements for comprehensiveness compared to those in urban areas, where other specialties may be available.

Core value of person-centredness

Africa has a diverse culture characterized by different languages, beliefs, and ways of living. This diversity exists within and between countries and regions of the continent. Despite this diversity, the consultation process within Africa begins with a rich greeting exploring the general feelings of the patient. More often than not, the patient expresses their 'reason for encounter', fears, expectations, and concerns during the greeting. What matters to the person or patient during the consultation is commonly expressed during the greeting. People feel happy and satisfied if this greeting is taken seriously by the providers. If this opportune moment of the consultation is missed, it is unlikely for the family physician to be patient-centred, as many patients are unlikely to voluntarily express their agenda. The doctor's agenda instead of the patient's agenda then becomes the main driver of the consultation, undermining the achievements of an effective and successful consultation.

Core value of family orientation

African societies attach great importance to family. Almost every patient has a significant family attachment, and this has implications on their presentation and care plan. Most patients come for a consultation accompanied by one or more family members. The family members are always interested in knowing what is happening and what is going to be done. The family as a whole sometimes has its own ideas, expectations, concerns, and fears. These should be recognized by the family physician and considered during information gathering, clinical reasoning, and care plan.

Core value of cultural identity

Despite globalization and other changes in the world, African societies still hold onto their culture. People feel respected and valued when their family doctor talks to them in their local language and demonstrates understanding of their ways of living. This makes it easy to establish a doctor–patient relationship that is likely to endure over time, promoting relational continuity. African communities are protective of their culture, and family physicians should acknowledge this attribute. Therefore, awareness and respect for patients' culture facilitates collaboration and shared decision-making during the consultation.

Core value of advocacy

Africa is home to 1.5 billion people and bears 20% of the global disease burden, coupled with the lowest levels of low human resources for health.[10,11] The region has several fragile states characterized by conflict and natural and human-caused disasters.[12] Most health systems are weak and unable to provide the necessary services to the populations.[13] Dictatorial governments are common, and the existing democracies are weak. Therefore, family physicians should engage with governments and relevant bodies and agencies for health systems to advocate for strengthening to improve performance and resilience. In most countries, the poverty levels are unacceptably high, with the poor being more vulnerable to disease and lacking access to care. Family physicians in Africa spend significant energy and time advocating for better and equitable healthcare for their patients, families, and communities.

Core value of community orientation

The diversity of communities in Africa requires an understanding of the unique needs of communities. Family physicians use their experience from consultations with individual patients to understand the common conditions among the population served. They work with the communities to make a community diagnosis. African family physicians have to understand the core functions of both primary care and essential public health services.[14,15] Such understanding helps them to provide services that are responsive to the needs of the communities served.

Core value of compassion

In SSA, family medicine is not a well-known or a prestigious specialty. Therefore, most of the family physicians chose the family medicine career out of compassion to provide quality care, particularly to vulnerable populations and communities. This compassion to care for the people is maintained and, in some way, drives all the other values in an effort to provide quality care. Family physicians fill practice gaps in facilities where there are no specialists. They work in rural and remote areas where no other specialists want to go.

They play a significant role in the epidemic response, for example, for COVID-19,[16] Ebola, and other haemorrhagic fevers, with most of these associated with high risk of death.

IMPLICATIONS AND APPLICATIONS

Family medicine curricula development and formulation of research agenda should be guided by these core values. As family medicine takes root in undergraduate medical education and evolvement of family medicine content in postgraduate education, understanding the core values is instrumental for improving social accountability of health profession training institutions.

Most countries in SSA do not have clearly documented family medicine training outcomes for their programmes. As countries strive to develop training outcomes to ensure uniformity among training institutions in their countries, core values will guide the process, as well as inform some of the outcomes.

As family medicine develops across SSA countries, there will be a need to focus on current global recommended assessment approaches and methods. Such approaches currently recommended include use of entrustable professional activities (EPAs).[17] The core values of family medicine can guide the development of some EPAs in the region.

Family physicians in Africa continue to struggle in defining their identity. This is because of the unclear description of their roles given that they work in an environment with another long-known general practitioner who has only one year of internship with no postgraduate training. A clear understanding of the family medicine core values will make a significant contribution towards defining family medicine and the identity of family physicians.

These core values should inform continuous professional development (CPD) content for family physicians working in the African region. This makes the CPD activities and efforts responsive to the needs of the family physicians in an attempt to serve their communities better.

Primary care research in SSA is still in its infancy.[18] However, it is steadily developing as evidenced by increase in the number of publications.[19,20] The core values of family medicine will greatly guide the development of the primary care research agenda, so researchers in primary care need to be familiar with these core values.

National and sub-national health policies in most countries in SSA are based on PHC, focusing on primary care as the main mode of service delivery.[21] Unfortunately, primary care is understood differently in different countries and is sometimes confused with PHC. The core values of family medicine, a primary care specialty if well understood by policymakers, can greatly inform proper and appropriate policy formulation.

CONCLUSION

Family medicine core values have been evolving in Africa with the development of the discipline. There are different family medicine practice models across the SSA region, but the values and principles appear to be the same. These values are embedded within the African cultural context within which most family physicians were born, grew, nurtured, studied, and are working. These core values help family physicians focus on patients, families and communities, and their needs, providing holistic care with an enduring doctor–patient relationship. This gives family medicine as a specialty, and family physicians as specialist practitioners, a unique identity and definition.

REFERENCES

1. Govender I, Omole O. Family medicine as a discipline in South Africa: Historical perspectives. *J Coll Med S Afr* 2023;1(1):3.
2. Udonwa N, Ariba A, Yohanna S, et al. Family medicine in West Africa: Progress, milestones, and challenges so far in Nigeria (1980–2010). *Niger J Fam Pr* 2011;1(2):1–9.
3. Mash R, Van Breevoort D, Makwero M, et al. Education for primary health care in Africa. *Afr J Prim Health Care Fam Med* 2023;15(1):4034.
4. Von Pressentin KB, Besigye I, Mash R, et al. The state of family medicine training programmes within the primary care and family medicine education network. *Afr J Prim Health Care Fam Med* 2020;12(1).
5. Besigye IK, Makasa M, Makwero M, et al. Next steps for the East, Central and Southern Africa College of Family Physicians (ECSA-CFP). *Afr J Prim Health Care Fam Med* 2024;16(1):1–2.
6. Downing R. African family medicine. *J Am Board Fam Med* 2008;21(2):169–70.
7. Reid S. The African family physician. *S Afr Fam Pract* 2007;49(9):3.
8. Mash R, Reid S. Statement of consensus on family medicine in Africa. *Afr J Prim Health Care Fam Med* 2010;2(1):1–4.
9. Ahmat A, Okoroafor SC, Kazanga I, et al. The health workforce status in the WHO African region: Findings of a cross-sectional study. *BMJ Global Health* 2022;7(Suppl 1):e008317.
10. Niohuru I. Disease burden and mortality. In: Niohuru I, ed. Healthcare and Disease Burden in Africa: The Impact of Socioeconomic Factors on Public Health. Cham: Springer International Publishing 2023:35–85.
11. Willcox ML, Peersman W, Daou P, et al. Human resources for primary health care in sub-Saharan Africa: Progress or stagnation? *Hum Res Health* 2015;13(1):76. https://doi.org/10.1186/s12960-015-0073-8
12. Dunne P, Tian N. Conflict and Fragile States in Africa: African Development Bank Abidjan, 2017.
13. World Health Organization. Health Systems in Africa: Community Perceptions and Perspectives: The Report of a Multi-Country Study, 2012.
14. World Health Organization. Primary health care measurement framework and indicators: Monitoring health systems through a primary health care lens. Web Annex: Technical Specifications, 2022.
15. Centre for Disease Control. The 10 Essential Public Health Services: CDC, 2020 [Available from: https://www.cdc.gov/public-health-gateway/php/about/index.html accessed 12 Dec 2024]
16. Ray S, Mash R. Innovation in primary health care responses to COVID-19 in Sub-Saharan Africa. *Prim Health Care Res Dev* 2021;22:e44.

17. Ten Cate O. Nuts and bolts of entrustable professional activities. *J Grad Med Educ* 2013;5(1):157–8. https://doi.org/10.4300/jgme-d-12-00380.1

18. Von Pressentin KB, Mash R, Ray SC, et al. Identifying research gaps and priorities for African family medicine and primary health care. *Afr J Prim Health Care Fam Med* 2024;16(1):4534.

19. Mash RJ, Von Pressentin K. Family practice research in the African region 2020–2022. *Afr J Prim Health Care Fam Med* 2024;16(1):4329.

20. Von Pressentin KB, Kaswa R, Murphy S, et al. A review of published research in the South African family practice – A clarion call to action. *S Afr Fam Pract* 2023;65(4).

21. World Health Organisation. Report on the Review of Primary Health Care in the African Region WHO Regional Office, Africa: WHO, 2008 [Available from: https://iris.who.int/bitstream/handle/10665/365669/9290231262-eng.pdf accessed 17 Dec 2024]

CHAPTER 4

Exploring core values in family medicine in the Asia Pacific Region

Sairat Noknoy, Leilanie Nicodemus, Harry H.X. Wang, Machiko Inoue, and Johanna Lynch

REGIONAL DESCRIPTION

The Asia Pacific is one of the seven regions of the World Organization of Family Doctors (WONCA). The healthcare landscape in the Asia Pacific region (APR) is complex and diverse, with substantial variations in accessibility, quality, and service delivery across different health systems. In recent decades, the APR has made considerable progress in expanding healthcare access and improving health outcomes.

The APR comprises 38 countries (Figure 4.1), of which only 17 are members of WONCA, with 24 Member Organisations (MOs), as some countries have more than one. Member countries encompass all the advanced economies: Australia, Hong Kong Special Administrative Region or SAR (HK), Japan, the Republic of Korea (South Korea), New Zealand (NZ), and Singapore. Some countries have yet to establish national-level professional organizations that hold membership in WONCA: Brunei, Kiribati, Laos, Marshall Islands, Nauru, Nepal, North Korea, Palau, Papua New Guinea, Samoa, Solomon Islands, Timor-Leste, Tonga, Tuvalu, and Vanuatu. Most have emerging markets and developing economies or are Pacific Island countries. Table 4.1 outlines demographics of the WONCA member countries.

DOI: 10.1201/9781003542353-4

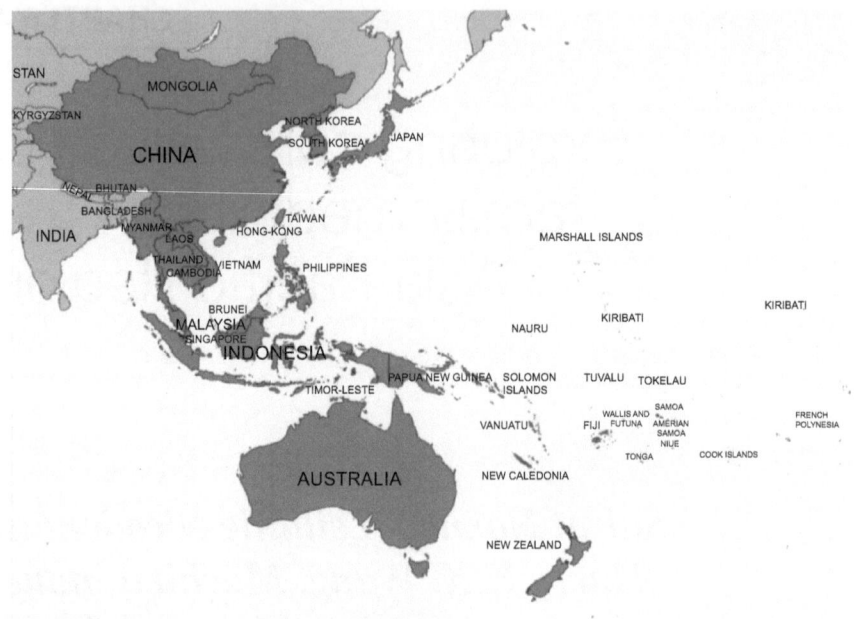

FIGURE 4.1 Map of the Asia Pacific region.

Source: Map created with Mapchart.net

Sixteen of the countries in the APR are defined as high-income, 9 as upper-middle, and 12 are low-middle-income. North Korea is the only low-income country in the region.[1] In general, lower-income countries face a high burden of disease because of limited access to quality healthcare, poor infrastructure, and high rates of poverty and malnutrition, which contribute to the spread of infectious diseases and suboptimal management of long-term conditions.[2]

APR has a diverse spectrum of environments, cultures, languages, and religions. Population size ranges from 700,000 (Macao SAR, China) to 1.4 billion (Mainland China). The average urbanization rate among WONCA member countries is 72%, with nearly two-thirds with a rate above 60%. Population density is particularly high in Macao, HK, and Singapore, with 100% urbanization, whereas other countries are more rural – the urbanization rate for Myanmar is 32%, and Vietnam and the Philippines are both under 50%. Unemployment also varies across the region, with the highest rates in Mongolia and lowest rates in Thailand and Vietnam.

On average, life expectancy at birth in the APR has grown steadily due to advancements in living standards, nutrition, and healthcare accessibility. The average life expectancy across MOs' health systems is 77.8 years. Macao and Japan have the highest life expectancy, exceeding 84 years, followed by

TABLE 4.1 WONCA Member Country Profiles

Country	Population in Millions[a]	Urban %[b]	Unemployment %[b]	GDP per Capita, USD[b]	Income Group[b]	Physicians per 1000 People[b]	Life Expectancy[b]	Life Expectancy (F)[b]	Life Expectancy (M)[b]	Population Age ≥65 (% total)[b]	Number GPs[a]	GPs per 1000 People
Australia	26.45	87	3.7	61,583.9	HIC	4.1	83	85	81	19.5	45,513	1.72
China	1422.58	65	4.7	12,175.2	UMIC	2.4	79	81	76	15.8	Unknown	Unknown
HK	7.54	100	3.9	43,573	HIC	1.3	84	87	81	21	12,000	1.6
Macao	0.68	100	2.2	59,602.4	HIC	1.6	85	88	83	13	Unknown	Unknown
Taiwan*[c]	23.42	76.9	3.48	32,404.3	HIC	–	80.23	83.28	76.63	18.3	Unknown	Unknown
Fiji	0.92	59	4.3	5,736.8	UMIC	0.8	68	70	66	7.6	Unknown	Unknown
Indonesia	282.19	59	3.4	4,192.6	UMIC	0.7	68	70	66	8.3	145,493	0.52
Japan	124.37	92	2.6	36,990.3	HIC	2.6	84	87	81	31.7	519	0.0042
South Korea	51.75	81	2.6	34,121	HIC	2.5	83	86	80	19.5	35,914	0.69
Malaysia	35.13	79	3.9	11,429.6	UMIC	2.2	76	79	74	8.6	924	0.026
Mongolia	3.43	69	6.1	4,456.5	UMIC	3.9	73	77	68	6.1	Unknown	Unknown
Myanmar	54.13	32	2.8	1,177.8	LMIC	0.8	67	70	64	8.3	Unknown	Unknown
NZ	5.17	87	3.7	41,766.9	HIC	3.5	83	84	81	18.8	6,478	1.25
Philippines	114.89	48	2.2	3,745.7	LMIC	0.8	72	74	70	6.3	Unknown	Unknown
Singapore	5.79	100	3.5	65,422.5	HIC	2.4	83	85	81	14.1	7,920	1.37
Thailand	71.70	54	0.9	6,393.9	UMIC	0.9	80	84	75	16.1	Unknown	Unknown
Vietnam	100.35	39	1.6	3760.4	LMIC	0.8	75	79	70	10	Unknown	Unknown

Key: GDP = gross domestic product; USD = United States dollars; LMIC = low-middle-income country; UMIC = upper-middle-income country; HIC = high-income country; F = female; M = male; GP = general practitioner; HK = Hong Kong SAR; Macao = Macao SAR; South Korea = the Republic of Korea; NZ = New Zealand.

Sources: [a]World Health Organization, https://www.who.int/; [b]World Bank, https://dataank.worldbank.org/; [c] (*Taiwan only) Statista, https://www.statista.com/

HK, Singapore, NZ, South Korea, and Australia, where life expectancy is 83 years or above. In Myanmar, Fiji, and Indonesia, life expectancy is below 70 years. Overall, women have higher life expectancy than men across all the health systems. The most pronounced gap is observed in Thailand, Vietnam, and Mongolia, where women have a projected life expectancy nine years longer than their male counterparts, compared to a gap of only four years in NZ and Indonesia.

Many countries are experiencing rapid population ageing, which reflects the success of healthcare and economic, educational, and social development over the last few decades. Japan and HK are the most aged societies, with 31.7% and 21% of their populations aged 65 years and over, respectively. The proportion of people in this age bracket is approaching 20% in South Korea, Australia, and NZ and is less than 10% in Mongolia, Philippines, Fiji, Indonesia, Myanmar, and Malaysia, It is projected that by 2050, the proportion of older people will be particularly large in South Korea, HK, and Japan, where over one-third of the population will be 65 and over. Health systems with a higher share of older people face greater challenges of long-term conditions such as arthritis, dementia, and cardiovascular disease that contribute significantly to higher levels of disability.[3]

The number of physicians varies considerably across the MO countries (mean = 1.96 per 1000 people). In six health systems (Indonesia, Fiji, Myanmar, Philippines, Vietnam, Thailand), the number of physicians is below 1.0 per 1000. Australia, Mongolia, and NZ have the highest per capita, at 4.1, 3.9, and 3.5 per 1000, respectively.[4] However, no data are available on the number of general practitioners/family physicians in most of the countries (see Table 4.1).

There are significant differences among healthcare systems in the region. Some countries embrace the concept of first-contact care and gatekeeping. In contrast, others adopt an approach that allows competition between primary care and specialist care, where it is common to bypass the first level of care to seek care at specialized departments in hospitals. This may increase the treatment burden due to fragmented, specialist-driven healthcare.[5] Gatekeeping is well established in NZ and Macao, whereas in Japan and the Philippines it is absent at the primary care level. A dual system is also common in the region. For example, in HK and Indonesia, people are free to choose between the public and private systems for healthcare, depending on their ability to pay. A universal single-payer insurance system has been adopted in South Korea, where every citizen must be enrolled in the National Health Insurance Service. There has been a growing emphasis on strengthening family medicine education and training to enhance primary care capacity and referral systems, while optimizing multidisciplinary team-based disease management in most health systems in the APR.

PROCESSES

The fundamental values of family medicine in the APR were examined through two lenses: statements from MOs and personal insights. Three methods were applied.

First, we reviewed the documents of WONCA APR MOs.[6] A dataset had previously been compiled for this project on the available vision, mission, and core values from 19 MOs' websites. This was augmented between March and July 2024 as further information was gathered using direct communication. Content analysis was used to organize and interpret the collected information, followed by thematic analysis to identify recurring themes and core values. All project team members reviewed and discussed the analysis to reach a consensus.

Second, a workshop was held to brainstorm family medicine's core values and meaning from family physicians' perspectives at the WONCA APR Conference, Singapore, in August 2024. Thirty-seven family physicians participated, representing China, Japan, Taiwan, the Philippines, Indonesia, Malaysia, Thailand, Myanmar, Singapore, Fiji, Australia, and NZ. Two key questions were used to prompt discussion:

'What inspires you as a family physician?' (97 written responses)
'Why do we need family doctors?' (91 written responses)

They also indicated their top three core values through Mentimeter, answering:

'What are the most important core values for you?'

Participants gave consent for their responses to be collected and collated. They wrote their answers to the first two questions on sticky notes and then reflected verbally with the group. Responses from 28 participants (GP1–GP28) were collected for the analysis. The third question was addressed through interactive voting to allow real-time aggregation of the most important core values identified by participants. The collected words were displayed in word cloud images.

Lastly, data from the two sources were triangulated to look for overarching themes and shared values of family medicine in the APR.

FINDINGS

The findings from this exploration are presented in three sections.

Core values of the WONCA APR MOs

A thematic analysis of core values outlined on 19 WONCA APR MO documents revealed 11 themes (Table 4.2), with trustworthy, high-quality care being a shared consensus among all MOs.

TABLE 4.2 Summary Findings From WONCA APR Member Organizations' Vision, Mission, and Core Value Statements

	Core Values Theme	Examples of Key Words and Phrases	Member Organizations	N
1.	Trustworthy (high-quality standards, competent, compassionate, ethical)	Ensure high-quality healthcare/promote the highest standard in general practice/strengthen service capabilities for general practitioners/improve professional competence/competent to provide a greater part of medical care/trustworthy primary care/raise primary medical care and family medicine standards/skilled and confidence/provide excellent healthcare/well-trained family physicians/distinguished/advancement/accountable/integrity/high-valued/compassionate/doctors who are not only skilled but who have confidence, commitment, and passion/building a caring society/ethical	ACRRM, RACGP, CSGP, SMEA-GP, FCGP, HKCFP, ISTFM, IAFP, JPCA, KAFM, AFPM, FMSA, MMA-GPS, RNZCGP, FAMed, PAFP, CFPS, CTAFM, GPFPT	19
2.	Generalism/ comprehensive care	Comprehensive/in all areas of care (including aged care, mental health, preventive care, rehabilitative and treatment, elderly, and end of life)/all health problems and diseases of people/see every stage of life (regardless of age, primary care for all age groups, lifetime health management/competent to provide the greater part of medical care/generalist medical practitioners/it is essential to have a doctor who can consult with about anything	ACRRM, RACGP, CSGP, SMEA-GP, FCGP, ISTFM, IAFP, JPCA, KAFM, AFPM, FMSA, FAMed, PAFP, CTAFM, GPFPT	15
3.	Multi-perspectivity/ holistic care	Multi-perspectivity/holistic/care towards patient, family, and community as a whole/interconnectedness of all things/art and science of medicine/bio-psycho-social model/can consult about anything	CSGP, JPCA, FMSA, RNZCGP, FAMed, PAFP, CFPS, CTAFM, GPFPT	9
4.	Cultural respect, diversity and inclusion	Culturally effective care/Aboriginal and Torres Strait Islander health/incorporate traditional Māori values/diversity and inclusion/ choice of Filipino families/health of the people of Malaysia/ irrespective of race, creed, or religion/regardless of age, race, and religion	RACGP, AFPM, FMSA, RNZCGP, FAMed, PAFP	6

(Continued)

TABLE 4.2 (Continued)

	Core Values Theme	Examples of Key Words and Phrases	Member Organizations	N
5.	Interconnected-relational (coordinated, collaborative, continuous)	Coordination/collaboration/continuous medical system/interconnectedness of all things and interrelationship with people/doctor–patient–family relationship/lifetime management through family doctors/foster solidarity among members, other specialties, and organisations/building a caring society and a united nation	JPCA, KAFM, AFPM, FMSA, RNZCGP, FAMed, PAFP, CTAFM, GPFPT	9
6.	Contextualized (person-centred, family and community oriented)	Individual need/personalised care/person-centred/patient-centred care is at the heart of every GP/put people's health at centre/patient- and family-centred/examining patient from multiple perspectives/values human dignity and respect for all people/families/family-centred/family-based/principle of family medicine/examining family and living background/the broader community/serving the community in every corner/examining the community/community-oriented health system/community- and population-based practice	ACRRM, RACGP, CSGP, FCGP, ISTFM, IAFP, JPCA, KAFM, AFPM, FMSA, RNZCGP, FAMed, PAFP, CTAFM, GPFPT	15
7.	Longitudinal/continuous	Lifetime health management through family doctors/continuing medical care/continuous	ACRRM, JPCA, KAFM, AFPM, FAMed, PAFP, CTAFM, GPFPT	8
8.	Primary healthcare foundation (backbone, accessible, first contact, primary care, community- and population-based)	The backbone of the country's health system/trustworthy primary care/primary contact/accessible/grassroots/universal healthcare/services for all/serving the community in every corner/essential to have a doctor nearby/lifetime management through a family doctor/maintains the health of nation's rural and remote communities/primary healthcare system/supported by community medicine and public health/leader responsible for community health/community- and population-based practice	ACCRM, RACGP, CSGP, FCGP, ISTFM, IAFP, JPCA, KAFM, AFPM, FMSA, RNZCGP, FAMed, PAFP, CTAFM, GPFPT	15

(Continued)

TABLE 4.2 (Continued)

	Core Values Theme	Examples of Key Words and Phrases	Member Organizations	N
9.	Improved health for all (equitable healthcare and sustainable)	Improve the health of all citizens, improve the health and wellbeing of all people/advocate for the health and wellbeing of the population in the nation/put people's health at the centre/happy and healthy life/improve health outcomes/health equity/equitable care/reduced inequality/providing rural and remote people with excellent healthcare/improving health services continuously at the grassroots/Aboriginal and Torres Strait Islander health sustainable servicers/economically viable	ACRRM, RACGP, CSGP, FCGP, ISTFM, IAFP, JPCA, KAFM, AFPM, MMA-GPS, RNZCGP, CFPS	12
10.	Health promotion/prevention	Health promotion/preventive care/not only sick people but also healthy people/health literacy among the population and people participation	RACGP, JPCA, KAFM, AFPM, FMSA, GPFPT	6
11.	Specialized	Specialist registration/primary care is the speciality of doctors/family medicine specialists/pertain family medicine specialist certification	ACRRM, JPCA, KAFM, AFPM, FMSA, PAFP, FAMed, PAFP, CTAFM, GFFPT	10

Trustworthiness was identified through the following characteristics: high-quality standards, accountability, integrity, competence, compassion, and ethics, which were vital to ensure service credibility. This was highlighted by the example of the Philippines Academy of Family Physicians (PAFP) with the vision 'To be the physician of choice of Filipino families'[7] and the Korean Academy of Family Medicine's (KAFM's) mission statement 'Trustworthy primary care, healthier people'.[8]

Generalism and comprehensiveness underscore the competency to provide care across all areas, including aged care, mental health, preventive care, rehabilitation, and end-of-life support. A generalist is well rounded, capable of addressing health needs at every stage of life and consulting about any issues. The Japan Primary Care Association (JPCA) emphasizes this in their vision, 'Comprehensive medical care for a healthy and happy life', and mission statement, 'We provide comprehensive medical care that is close to you and that you can consult about anything'.[9]

Holistic care, or a multi-perspectivity approach in family medicine, sees the interconnectedness of various aspects of health and ensures comprehensive support for individuals. The holistic approach provides care to the person, family, and community as an interconnected unit. This value was documented in the Malaysian Family Medicine Specialist Association's (FMSA's) vision, 'Caring towards the patient, his/her family and community as a whole', and the PAFP's mission to 'Advance holistic care for individuals, families and communities'.[10] This value embodies a bio-psycho-social model of medicine and the integration between art and science, the blended component of the whole, also stated in the College of Family Physicians of Singapore's (CFPS's) mission, 'To advance the Art and Science of Medicine'.[11]

Cultural respect, diversity, and inclusion are components of the multi-perspective and holistic approach. These values underline that family physicians must cultivate cultural sensitivity and be capable of recognizing the unique traditional values and beliefs of diverse communities, regardless of age, race, creed, or religion: 'Family Medicine specialists dedicated to providing holistic, accessible, continuous, comprehensive, family-centred, coordinated, compassionate and culturally effective health care' by the Foundation for Family Medicine Educators (FAMed) and the PAFP.[7]

The interconnectedness and interrelationships of all things underscore the necessity of coordination and collaboration to enable continuous and comprehensive care. It also highlights the relationships between individuals, families, and healthcare providers, as well as the doctor–patient and family relationship, which are crucial for health management. The Royal New Zealand College of General Practitioners (RNZCGP) elaborates on respect and collaboration: 'A commitment to practice respect and collaboration by acknowledging the interconnectedness of all things and inter-relationships with people'.[12] Collaboration is essential to promote a united caring society, as highlighted in the mission of the General Practitioners/Family Physicians Association of Thailand (GPFPT): 'Foster solidarity among members and physicians of other specialties', and the FMSA's mission: 'to build a caring society and a united Malaysian nation.'[10]

Contextualized care, emphasizing a person-centred approach and prioritizing the wellbeing of individuals within their family and community contexts, was underscored in most MOs' statements. Personalized care is the cornerstone for effective care, as each person's needs are unique and influenced by personal circumstances, family dynamics, and the broader community environment. Context-based practice addresses interconnected factors to ensure tailored care for how they live, work, and interact with communities. The Chinese Taipei Association of Family Medicine (CTAFM) states in their core values: 'Based on the bio-psycho-social model, we provide comprehensive, continuous, coordinated, accessible and accountable medical services and establish a person-centred, family-based and community-oriented healthcare system'.[13]

Longitudinal and continuous care addresses the importance of ongoing health management throughout a patient's life. It fosters a doctor–patient relationship that supports proactive prevention, monitoring, and treatment for overall wellbeing over time. This was emphasized by the Australian College of Rural and Remote Medicine (ACRRM), 'The general practitioner is the doctor with core responsibility for providing comprehensive and continuing medical care to individuals, families and the broader community'[14] and also by the KAFM, *Lifetime Health Management through a Family Doctor*.[8]

Primary healthcare (PHC) is the foundation of the health and wellbeing of a country's population, comprising the integration of the backbone of primary care services and public health functions. Trustworthy primary care provides first-contact medical services at the grassroots level and strengthens universal healthcare, ensuring health for all. This was highlighted in the Fiji College of General Practitioners' (FCGP's) vision: 'A primary health care system which delivers quality medical care according to individual need'. The community-oriented population-based practice principle was adopted by the GPFPT and by the Indonesian Society of Teachers and Family Medicine (ISTFM), 'Primary care physicians in Indonesia consists of physicians who consistently apply principles of family medicine, supported by community and public health and able to lead primary health care in high-quality services and care'.

The goal of the PHC is enabling health for all. Fair distribution of resources and health services are essential means towards this path, as echoed by

RNZCGP's vision: 'To improve health outcomes and reduce health inequalities'.[12] The Academy of Family Physicians of Malaysia (AFPM) also reiterated health for all: 'To advance the art and science of medicine for the general benefit of mankind irrespective of race, creed or religion and to improve the health and well-being of individuals, families and communities'.[10] Likewise, population wellbeing is highlighted by the Royal Australian College of General Practitioners' (RACGP's) mission: 'to improve the health and well-being of all people in Australia',[15] emphasizing the meaning of health, which is not only the absence of disease but a state of complete physical, mental, and social well-being.

Commitment through these values enables sustainable and economically viable systems, led by ACRRM's mission: 'We are committed to delivering sustainable, high-quality health services to rural and remote communities'.[14] Health promotion and preventive services are crucial for family practitioners, highlighted by KAFM: 'Family Physicians are doctors who protect the health of the entire family'.[8] JPCA holds a similar core value: 'Primary is a service that sees not only sick people but also healthy people from infants to elderly. It's essential to have a doctor (general practitioner/family doctor) nearby who can consult about anything at no time, not only disease but also preventive medicine'.[9]

Acknowledgement of the unique skills and wisdom of family medicine is essential to ensure high-quality healthcare. Family physicians play a vital role in the healthcare system, commanding a broad range of knowledge and skills to provide care for all age groups with diverse backgrounds. Specific training, mentoring, and certification in generalism ensures that family physicians are prepared with the knowledge and skills essential for the diverse health needs of individuals and families. This expertise allows family physicians to navigate complex health issues effectively. The need for a system to maintain family physicians' capacity was highlighted by many MOs through their mission, as CTAFM affirmed: 'to promote the development of a family physician specialist system'.[13]

In summary, the core values of family medicine, articulated by MOs in the APR, emphasize trustworthy, high-quality services by compassionate family physicians. These specialists are competent, well-rounded practitioners who excel in holistic care, integrating diverse perspectives to provide comprehensive and coordinated services tailored to individual, family, community, and cultural circumstances. Grounded in the principles of PHC, family medicine prioritizes accessible primary care services that are integrated into community population–oriented practices throughout their lifetime, focus on marginalized populations to bridge the equity gap, and embrace preventive measures to build sustainable systems and health for all.

Values expressed by family physicians brainstorming workshop

Family physicians' responses to the discussion prompts were summarized into three core values:

1. **Patient-centred holistic care**: A comprehensive approach that views patients as whole individuals, not just their medical conditions. This value emphasizes treating the complete person by considering health's physical, emotional, and social aspects while building strong, trusting personal relationships between healthcare providers and patients through empathy and compassion.
2. **Family and community integration of healthcare delivery**: Recognizing the vital role of family support systems and community connections in patient outcomes. This approach focuses on strengthening family relationships, promoting community health education, and ensuring healthcare services are accessible and equitable for entire populations.
3. **Preventive and sustainable healthcare**: A proactive healthcare model emphasizing prevention, early intervention, and long-term wellness. This value incorporates lifelong learning, adaptability to individual needs, and cost-effective strategies.

As summarized in the word cloud in Figure 4.2, when asked 'What inspires you as a family physician?', most participants responded that their inspiration was because of the variety, caring nature of the work, their patients, and compassion. Others mentioned that their patients inspire them, the caring relationship, service to others, and the whole-person approach. At the core is a focus on 'my patients' care,' emphasizing a holistic, compassionate approach that values the whole person and variety, not just their medical condition.

Their responses also highlight the importance of strong patient–provider relationships rooted in qualities like empathy, patience, and positive regard. It stresses the role of healthcare professionals in motivating, educating, and supporting patients and their families throughout their care journeys. Concepts like preventive care, lifelong learning, and adapting to individual needs underscore this model's proactive, personalized nature.

Beyond the clinical relationship, family physicians emphasized the value of connecting communities, promoting health and wellness, and addressing the bio-psycho-social factors that impact patient outcomes. Themes like equity, collaborative communication, and serving the broader population reflect a commitment to healthcare as a means of uplifting entire communities. Taken together, these family physicians described a profoundly human-centric vision of healthcare. It goes far beyond just medical treatment to focus on the overall wellbeing and quality of life of patients, their families, and the communities of which they are a part.

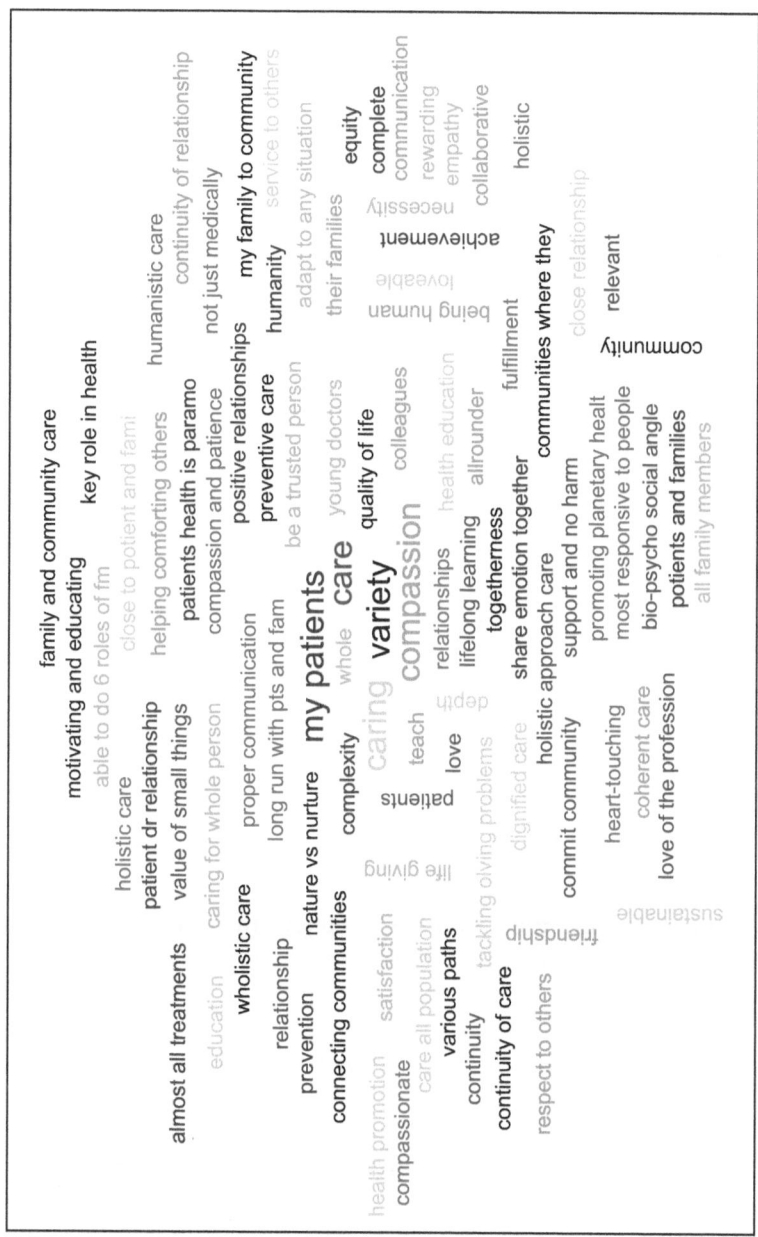

FIGURE 4.2 Word cloud presentation of responses to 'What inspires you as a family physician?'

As summarized in the word cloud in Figure 4.3, when asked 'Why do we need family physicians?' most responses focused on family and community medicine practice, managing patients' life courses, emphasizing preventive care, and taking a humanistic approach to healing. Their responses highlight various reasons why family physicians are essential in healthcare. Key themes include their depth of knowledge and ability to provide comprehensive, holistic, compassionate care that considers the whole person, not just their medical condition, and their perseverance to provide continuous care for patients and families, resulting in building trusting relationships.

Given this, family physicians serve as a consistent first point of contact for the people under their care and guide them through the healthcare system throughout their lives. Their understanding of the family and community context and ability to integrate care was also emphasized. Other benefits mentioned include accessibility, cost-effectiveness, preventive care focus, expertise in managing uncertainty and challenging life situations, and the role of family physicians as community leaders and advocates. These findings suggest we need family physicians because they can deliver humane, personalized healthcare that addresses the full spectrum of patient and community needs.

INSIGHTS AND INTEGRATION

To fully understand family medicine's core values, findings from individual family physicians' brainstorming workshops were triangulated with the findings from the review of MOs' documents. Notably, family physicians' perspectives gathered through face-to-face interactions in the workshop uncovered more subjective insights and a deeper appreciation for the humanistic aspects of family practice. These findings validated small things, such as the meaning of caring, usually uncountable but experienced and often overlooked in the scientific arena yet considered highly valued by family physicians: connection, sharing, togetherness, heart-touching, long-running relationships, understanding, and prevention, to name but a few. By synthesising the data from the two sources, we concluded with six key themes encapsulating family medicine practice's core values as follows:

1. **Wholehearted/deep holistic care – beyond medical and not fragmented care:**

The discipline looks at the whole picture, a combination of art and science, to understand the interconnection between the biomolecular level of pathophysiologic changes; personal experiences and wishes; and their relation to family, sociocultural, and community environment. Family physicians voiced their inspiration and need for the profession:

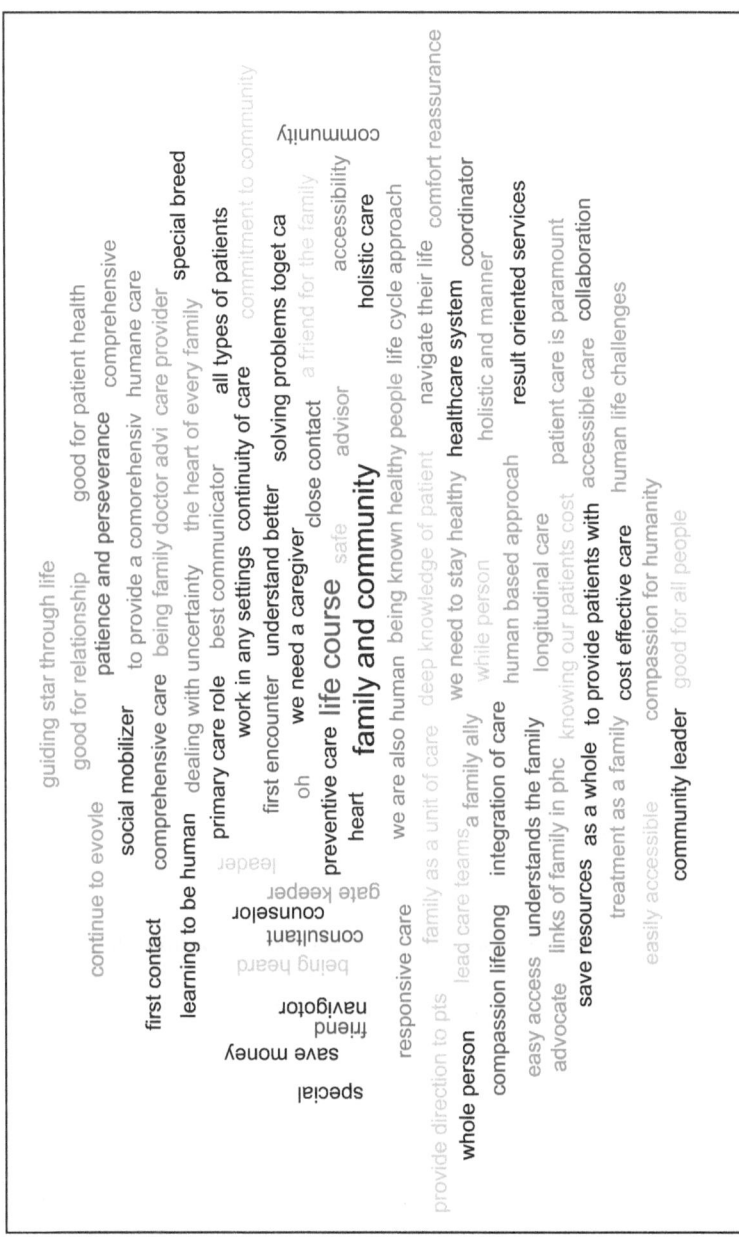

FIGURE 4.3 Word cloud presentation of responses to 'Why do we need family physicians?'

'Inspired by the bio-psycho-socio-cultural concept, holistic, comprehensive concepts, so does community-oriented' (GP14)

'Delivering holistic care, not fragmented health care' (GP19)

'Holistic medicine and care for patients – wholesome care for the whole family disregards of organs and age groups and gender – all spectrum of medical care' (GP 27).

A comprehensive approach to patient care, multi-perspectivity, or holistic care is key to the quality of care valued by family physicians as demonstrated by their responses:

'I want to give quality health care to my patients . . . I want to provide comprehensive care to them' (GP1)

'Comprehensive management' (GP15)

Moreover, the value of holistic medicine is not only about the dimension of care delivered but also how care is delivered, totally with compassion. The role of a family physician as a care provider, serving as a medium to deliver care, signifies this part:

'As family physician not just medically but be able to apply the roles of family physician' (GP2)

'Essence of being a doctor' (GP19)

2. **Compassionate, whole-of-life, high-quality care**: Compassion emerged as central when family physicians shared their inspiration for being in the profession (Figure 4.1). Trustworthiness was pronounced in MOs' statements, with five specifying compassion. Family physicians in the workshop voiced humanistic care, with compassion standing out:

'Shared understanding, passion, commitment, variety of problems' (GP1)

'Love, respect, service' (GP18)

'A physician with a heart, and the love for people' (GP2)

Compassion extends beyond the person to the community, by the nature of primary care:

'Helping people, comforting them, connecting people, being part of the community' (GP4)

'As the primary source of care when you don't know what to do with your problems, you can ask your family physician when you have a life-threatening illness. Even if it's not curable, family physicians can take care' (GP 6)

Family physicians are committed to providing high-quality care, adjusted to individual circumstances and integrated with compassion, voiced through both aspirations:

'I want to give quality health care to my patients' (GP1)
'Integrating our compassion' and the need for family physicians 'because FP delivers high-quality, compassionate, and cost-effective care' (GP28)

Caring for life goes beyond the medical part, making it complex and demanding various skills, and thus challenging. These, however, turned out to be the inspiration for family physicians, as verbalized:

'Complexity of patients and variety of backgrounds, problems, concerns, solutions, life' (GP6)
'I like different roles and variety of work' (GP23)

Their aspiration for continuous learning contributed to their competencies:

'Learning from others, both patients and professionals' (GP4)

Connecting and sharing knowledge with others empowers family physicians to grow their wisdom through their path, which is how family medicine grows as a unique and valued skill set and continues to evolve:

'Sense of connection to family physicians' community, fraternity . . . nurturing young family doctors' (GP12)
'We are life specialists; we continue to evolve' (GP27)

3. Continuous relationships – companions to help navigate safe and appropriate care: Witnessing the interconnectedness of all things, family physicians play an important role in connecting all the dots. In family practice, relationship building is the core of enabling effective care: the relationship between doctors and patients, multidisciplinary teams, other specialists, family and community workers, and related stakeholders. In relationships, communication was emphasized:

'Proper communication' (GP8)

Apart from coordinating needed services, connecting has a deep meaning, including comfort, companionship, and healing:

'For integrated care of patients' (GP11)
'Close and deep, patient-doctor relationship' (GP25)
'We need friends, we need people that we are familiar with' (GP5)

The enduring doctor–patient–family relationship that fosters trust and well-being across the lifespan was seen as very important:

'Continue the practice for the same family member' (GP12)
'Feel well seeing me in the long-term relationship' (GP20)

This value underscores the significant role of family physicians as lifelong health companions, navigating patients through life's journeys:

'Family doctors play a role as a guiding star to walk through the life journey of patients' (GP11)
'We need a lifelong companion for our health/we need an advisor for our health' (GP23)

4. **Family-focused care**: The importance of family and community was central in the responses to the question about why we need family physicians. The fundamental role of the family in healthcare delivery was recognized, viewing it as the basic unit of a healthy society. Physicians described how family dynamics significantly influence individual health outcomes, with functional families supporting patient management, while dysfunctional relationships can adversely affect health.

By establishing long-term relationships with families, family physicians position themselves as trusted partners to ensure the health and wellbeing of the family. Their scope of care extends beyond individual patients to the entire family, including extended family members and the broader community. This comprehensive approach allows them to deliver holistic care considering the interconnected nature of family health to society. This family-centred approach enables them to provide continuous, integrated care that benefits not just patients and families but the entire system:

'Realised that family can support the management of the patient, vice versa somehow the dysfunction of the family could affect the health condition, that's why I got inspired' (GP15)
'Functional, healthy, the family is the foundation of a healthy population, society and planet' (GP17)

5. **Welcoming, accessible, community-based care**: Family physicians transcend traditional medical care by serving as community health resources. They practice community-oriented primary care by examining and addressing health needs in every corner of their communities, enabling access to the marginalized, as seen in their responses:

'Working in regional, rural, remote' (GP6)
'Respond to lack of doctors deserted town, isolated island, for our patients' families' communities, symbols of community health' (GP12)

They serve as primary care providers, offering a broad range of services to sick and healthy individuals and ensuring lifetime health management through trusted relationships. They build lasting connections with patients, families, and the broader community through compassionate service and a continuous presence:

'First contact of care for the patients and holistic approach with the continuing of care from womb to tomb' (GP28)

With well-rounded competency, they welcome all, regardless of age, gender, social status, or the type of problem:

'First contact for any type of problem, compassionate docs who care for patients, family, community' (GP16)
'I get to see patients regardless of age, gender, social status' (GP19)
'Whatever he/she needs' (GP11)

The family physician's role is essential in optimizing patient outcomes through shared understanding and involvement in transformative care. By addressing individual and community health, family physicians uniquely position themselves as irreplaceable leaders in primary care:

'Because of the diversity of our knowledge and practice, we can channel our and patients to the best direction they need' (GP21)

Their commitment extends to community medicine and public health, working to protect and promote the health of defined populations. This population-based approach allows them to understand and respond to local health patterns while improving public health knowledge. Through this comprehensive approach, they contribute to community wellbeing:

'Care for patients and their families and the community where they live' (GP28)

6. **Preventive, competent, efficient services for the wellbeing of our planet**: Family physicians are key in providing preventive, high-quality, efficient healthcare that supports sustainable health systems:

'To save health care resources of patients, families, communities and countries' (GP11)

Family physicians are specialists in primary care, certified to deliver high standards of care and trusted by families as their doctor of choice. Their integration into community systems enables them to serve as accessible contact points for healthcare needs. They are the backbone of health systems, compassionate, well-rounded clinicians, enabling efficient and equitable care:

'Basic unit of the health care system' (GP1)
'Because FP delivers high quality, compassionate and cost-effective care' (GP17)

Their focus extends beyond treating illnesses to health promotion and disease prevention, ensuring healthier populations and conserving healthcare resources. Their practice integrates clinical expertise with community advocacy, fostering a healthcare environment:

'Allrounder benefits more people, preventive care, total satisfaction' (GP3)
'Having been involved with my city health promotion' (GP12)

The profession also appreciates simplicity and small things with a lasting impact. It advocates for safety and cost-effective healthcare:

'Medicine works best in context; meet patients where they are at holistic care affordable' (GP7)

With their commitment to excellence and respect, family physicians play a vital role in strengthening healthcare systems and evolving to meet the changing needs of their communities. They maintain system efficiency by prioritizing innovation and sustainability and advocating universal health coverage. This multi-layered approach ensures that family physicians remain central to individual health outcomes and broader public health initiatives. These values were stated as follows:

'Community commitment, professional integrity, future generation safety, ecosystem maintenance and protection of values' (GP22)

Furthermore, the value held by family physicians is not only what they believe but also what they experience:

'Feeling that we involve changing patients' lives' (GP24)
'Working with a community, a big change in prognosis' (GP7)

In conclusion, family medicine is a unique discipline with a distinct approach to caring for the whole person, family, and community; the emerging themes are indeed interconnected with holism.

IMPLICATIONS AND APPLICATIONS

The core values of family medicine emphasize the humanistic aspects of medical care, rooted in compassion and the importance of relationships. These values are vital for delivering holistic care that spans personal interactions to support families and communities throughout life, forming the foundation of high-quality care.

Family physicians are committed not only to individual patient care but also to the public good, grounded in the principles of primary healthcare. Their dedication to equitable healthcare and wellbeing is paired with a focus on sustainable health systems. Our findings resonate with WONCA's mission[16] and reflect the insights of Ian McWhinney,[17] who, in his early work, underscored the humanistic dimensions of medicine for individuals and families. These common findings are also reported in core values explored in other recent studies.[18-20] Our exploration of the core values within the APR family medicine community highlights the critical importance of community and public health orientation, especially in resource-limited settings.

Believing that our values are essential for achieving the health and wellbeing of populations prompts us to reflect on whether we are on the right path to success. A review of the mission statements of APR MOs reveals a strong commitment to enhancing quality standards of care and building practice capacity through education and training. Additionally, these organizations prioritize research and innovation, advocacy, professional recognition, and social and cultural integration, along with fostering regional and global collaboration. These strategic initiatives align closely with the values we uphold, suggesting that we are moving in a direction that supports our overarching goals for improved health outcomes.

This raises several important questions: Are our values recognized, accepted, and supported by the public and stakeholders? How can we effectively pursue our goals in alignment with these values? Are our values integrated into the country's value-based healthcare framework and measurement systems? Does the current system adequately support our values?

What adjustments are needed for our continued evolution? Additionally, what should we prioritize in our missions to ensure we achieve our objectives based on our core beliefs?

As family medicine experiences social and healthcare pressures, defining core values can help protect our work's heart. The initial exploration of core values described in this chapter will lead to further exploration in each member country and across the region as we work to support the critical role of family medicine in years to come. Clarifying core values will help individual practitioners, national MOs, university and postgraduate training, and wider national and international primary care leaders champion and protect the family doctor's work in their communities.

CONCLUSION

The exploration of core values of family medicine in the APR described a unified vision built on the unique trustworthy, culturally respectful, contextualized, longitudinal, and relational skills of family physicians. The core values were named as wholehearted and deep holistic care that goes beyond the medical and is not fragmented; compassionate, whole-of-life, high-quality care; continuous relationships that navigate towards safe and appropriate care; family-focused care; welcoming, accessible, and community-based care; and preventative, competent, efficient services for the wellbeing of the planet. We anticipate further exploration of how we can create meaningful impact based on the identified values and expand our collaboration to engage a broader community, thereby realising greater benefits in practice.

ACKNOWLEDGEMENTS

We would like to thank Associate Professor Liz Sturgiss from the School of Primary and Allied Health Care at Monash University for her contributions to the development on methods for exploring core values. We particularly thank Professor Karen Flegg, WONCA president, for her unwavering support. Furthermore, we extend our heartfelt thanks to the WONCA APR 2024 Singapore Organizing Committee and all family physicians who participated in the workshop; their engagement and insights were integral to the success of this exploration.

REFERENCES

1. The World Bank. World Bank Country and Lending Groups, 2025 [Available from: https://datahelpdesk.worldbank.org/knowledgebase/articles/906519-world-bank-country-and-lending-groups accessed Jan 2025]
2. OECD/WHO. Health at a Glance: Asia/Pacific 2024, Paris. Paris: OECD Publishing, 2024. https://doi.org/10.1787/51fed7e9-en

3. Kowal P, Hoang T, Ng N. Universal Health Coverage and Ageing in Developing Asia. Malaysia: Asia Development Bank, 2020:40.
4. Global Health Observatory. Explore a World of Health Data, Geneva: WHO 2024 [Available from: https://www.who.int/data/gho accessed Jan 2025]
5. Hu XJ, Wang HHX, Li YT, et al. Healthcare needs, experiences and treatment burden in primary care patients with multimorbidity: An evaluation of process of care from patients' perspectives. *Health Expect* 2022;25(1):203–13. https://doi.org/10.1111/hex.13363 [published Online First: 2021/09/30].
6. WONCA Global Family Doctor. Member Organizations: Asia Pacific region: WONCA, 2025 [accessed Jan 2025]
7. Philippine Academy of Family Physicians. About Us. Vision and Mission PAFP, 2024 [Available from: https://thepafp.org/ accessed Dec 2024]
8. Korean Academy of Family Medicine. What is family medicine? Seoul, 2024 [Available from: https://www.kafm.or.kr/about/introduce02_eng.php]
9. Japan Primary Care Association. General Medical Care for a Healthy and Happy Life Tokyo. Japan: JPCA, 2024 [Available from: https://www.primarycare-japan.com/about.htm accessed Dec 2024]
10. Family Medicine Specialist Association. About FMSA: FMSA, 2024 [Available from: https://fms-malaysia.org/about-fmsa/ accessed Dec 2024]
11. College of Family Physicians Singapore. College Mission, 2024 [Available from: https://www.cfps.org.sg/about-us/college-mission/ accessed Dec 2024]
12. Royal New Zealand College of General Practitioners. Te Rautaki Statement of Strategic Intent 2019–2024: RNZCGP, 2024:14.
13. Taiwan Association of Family Medicine. Mission, 2024 [Available from: https://www.tafm.org.tw/ehc-tafm/s/w/Mission/article/a1aec91c647d4d7ca8cc27dfc5afcd1e accessed Dec 2024]
14. Australian College of Rural and Remote Medicine. College Definition of General Practice: ACRRM, 2024 [Available from: https://www.acrrm.org.au/about-us/about-the-college/college-definition-of-general-practice accessed Dec 2024]
15. Royal Australian College of General Practitioners. About Us: RACGP, 2024 [Available from: https://www.racgp.org.au/the-racgp/about-us accessed Dec 2024]
16. WONCA. WONCA in Brief Bangkok, 2013 [Available from: http://www.globalfamilydoctor.com/AboutWonca/brief.aspx accessed Jul 2015]
17. McWhinney I. A Textbook of Family Medicine. Oxford, UK: Oxford University Press 1989.
18. Arvidsson E, Švab I, Klemenc-Ketiš Z. Core values of family medicine in Europe: Current state and challenges. *Fron Med* 2021;8:646353. https://doi.org/10.3389/fmed.2021.646353 [published Online First: 2021/03/13].
19. Lawson HJO, Nortey DNN. Core values of family physicians and general practitioners in the African context. *Front Med* 2021;8. https://doi.org/10.3389/fmed.2021.667144
20. Cubaka VK, Dyck C, Dawe R, et al. A global picture of family medicine: The view from a WONCA storybooth. *BMC Fam Pract* 2019;20(1):129. https://doi.org/10.1186/s12875-019-1017-5 [published Online First: 2019/09/14].

CHAPTER 5

Exploring core values in family medicine in the East Mediterranean

*Mona Osman, Faisal A. AlNaser,
Nagwa Nashat Hegazy,
and Wadeia Sharief*

REGIONAL DESCRIPTION

The WONCA Eastern Mediterranean Region (EMR) encompasses 22 countries spanning the Middle East, North Africa, and parts of South Asia (see Figure 5.1). Each country is characterized by diverse cultural, political, and socioeconomic landscapes.[1-3] The region is distinguished by its rich cultural heritage, strategic geopolitical significance, and stark contrasts in economic conditions, ranging from extreme wealth to profound poverty.[3] Home to 680 million people, the EMR accounts for 9% of the global population.[1] Unfortunately, armed conflicts affect 12 of its countries, and the region harbours 64% of the world's refugee population, underscoring the magnitude of its humanitarian challenges.[1,4]

The EMR of WONCA largely overlaps with the WHO-EMR countries, except for Pakistan and the inclusion of Algeria and South Sudan.[5,6] Within this region, 17 countries have established member organizations in WONCA EMR: Afghanistan, Algeria, Bahrain, Egypt, Iraq, Islamic Republic of Iran, Jordan, Kuwait, Lebanon, Libya, Morocco, Oman, Palestine, Qatar, Saudi Arabia, Syria, and the United Arab Emirates[6,7] (see Appendix).

DOI: 10.1201/9781003542353-5

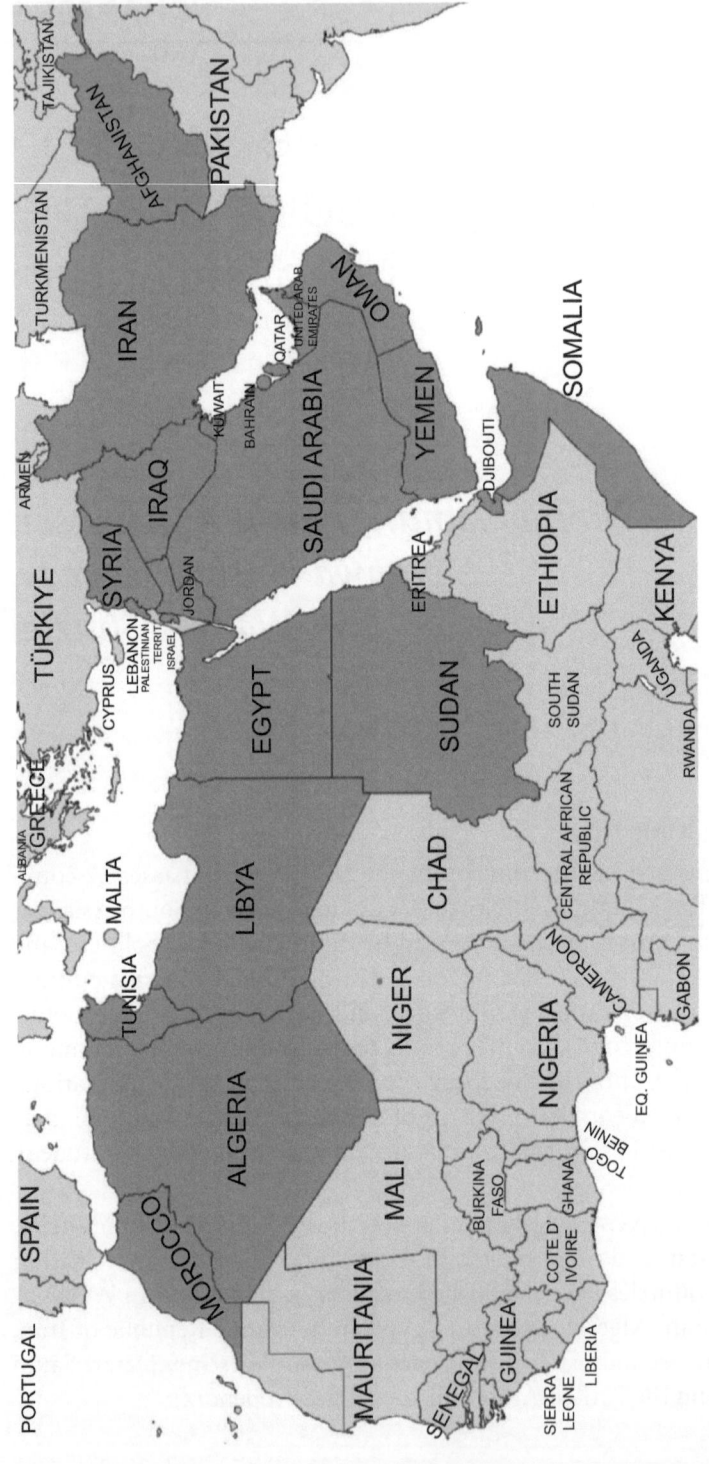

FIGURE 5.1 Map of the countries in East Mediterranean region.

Source: mapchart.net

The countries within the region exhibit significant variations in income levels, population size, and degree of urbanization.[8–10] Of these, six countries are classified as high income, four as upper middle income, seven as lower middle income, and six as low income (Table 5.1).[8] Egypt has the largest population in the region at 116 million, while Djibouti has the smallest with just over 1 million.[9,10] Afghanistan, Egypt, Somalia, Sudan, and South Sudan are notably more rural than the other countries in the region.[9,10] Arabic is the predominant native language across most of these countries, although languages such as French and English are widely spoken, reflecting the influence of past colonial histories.

TABLE 5.1 Characteristics of the Countries of WONCA EMR[8–10]

Country	Income Range	Total Population	Density (P/km²)	% Urban
Afghanistan	LIC	42,647,492	65	27
Algeria	UMIC	46,814,308	20	74
Bahrain	HIC	1,607,049	2115	≈100
Djibouti	LMIC	1,168,722	50	71
Egypt	LMIC	116,538,258	117	41
Iraq	UMIC	46,042,015	106	72
Islamic Republic of Iran	UMIC	91,567,738	56	73
Jordan	LMIC	11,552,876	130	84
Kuwait	HIC	4,934,507	277	92
Lebanon	LMIC	5,805,962	568	88
Libya	UMIC	7,381,023	4	77
Morocco	LMIC	38,081,173	85	67
Oman	HIC	5,281,538	17	93
Palestine	LMIC	5,495,443	913	83
Qatar	HIC	3,048,423	263	97
Saudi Arabia	HIC	33,962,757	16	92
Somalia	LIC	19,009,151	30	46
South Sudan	LIC	11,943,408	20	27
Sudan	LIC	50,448,963	29	35
Syria	LIC	24,672,760	134	53
Tunisia	LMIC	12,277,109	79	71
United Arab Emirates	HIC	11,027,129	132	82
Yemen	LIC	40,583,164	77	33

HIC: high-income country; UMIC: upper-middle-income country; LMIC: lower-middle-income country; LIC: low-income country.

ACCESS TO FAMILY MEDICINE

The EMR exhibits considerable diversity in its healthcare systems and access to family medicine.[11-13] Family medicine training programmes have been introduced in most countries of the region since 1979, starting with Lebanon, followed shortly by Bahrain, and later expanding across the region.[11,14,15] The establishment of the Arab Board of Family and Community Medicine Council (now the Scientific Council of Family Medicine) in 1986, as part of the Arab Board of Health Specializations, marked a significant milestone. This body, with membership from most Arab countries, aims to define standards for family medicine training in the Arab world.[16,17]

However, there remains a significant shortage of family physicians (FPs) in the EMR. It is estimated that 210,000 FPs need to be trained annually to achieve the recommended ratio of three FPs per 10,000 population.[18,19] The role and practice of FPs vary widely across the region.[15] In some countries, such as Bahrain, FPs act as gatekeepers, serving as the first point of entry into the healthcare system.[3,11] However, in others, particularly those with privatized healthcare systems such as Lebanon, specialized care dominates. In these settings, individuals can access specialists directly in both public and private sectors without a referral system.[17,20]

Access to family medicine in the EMR is shaped by disparities in health-care systems, economic development, political stability, and resources.[11-13] High-income countries in the region boast well-established family medicine programmes, supported by robust primary healthcare systems, modern facilities, and favourable policies.[11] In middle-income countries, access varies due to workforce shortages, uneven rural-urban distribution, and limited funding. Countries like Egypt and Jordan are making efforts to strengthen family medicine–based care models.[20,21] However, middle-income countries experiencing conflicts, such as Lebanon, face significant challenges because of their strained healthcare systems.[12]

In low-income and conflict-affected countries such as Afghanistan, Palestine, Sudan, and Syria, family medicine faces barriers, including fragile healthcare systems, inadequate infrastructure, limited training opportunities, and funding constraints.[11] Additionally, countries like Yemen, Somalia, South Sudan, and Djibouti lack well-established family medicine programmes, further limiting access to this vital specialty.[11]

PROCESSES

A mixed-methods approach was employed to gather data on the values, principles, vision, mission, and competencies of family medicine in the EMR. This involved a comprehensive literature review and an analysis of information from websites and social media platforms of various family medicine societies and associations. Key details regarding values, mission, vision, principles, and competencies in family medicine were extracted.

Additionally, a Google survey was distributed to representatives of family medicine societies/associations, WONCA EMR members, and the Scientific Council of Family Medicine at the Arab Board of Health Specializations. The survey aimed to capture their perceptions of family medicine values, implementation, and challenges within their respective countries. Responses were received from 15 countries: Afghanistan, Algeria, Bahrain, Egypt, Iraq, Jordan, Lebanon, Morocco, Oman, Palestine, Saudi Arabia, Sudan, Syria, Tunisia, and the United Arab Emirates.

A core values workshop was arranged for the WONCA EMR Family Medicine Congress in Amman, Jordan, October 2024. Unfortunately, an outbreak of conflict in the region disrupted travel, and the workshop was unable to go ahead.

FINDINGS

The definition, attributes, and functions of family medicine have been established since the specialty's inception in the region, drawing inspiration from American and European models.[14] Core values have been articulated across various family medicine training programmes. While countries in the region share many overlapping values and principles, these have been adapted to align with their unique healthcare systems and cultural contexts. These 14 key core values and principles specific to the EMR are (1) comprehensive care, (2) continuity of care, (3) patient-centred care, (4) compassionate care, (5) equity and access, (6) prevention and health promotion, (7) cultural sensitivity and respect for diversity, (8) community-oriented care, (9) advocacy, (10) resilience and adaptability, (11) collaboration and teamwork, (12) ethical practice and professionalism, (13) quality improvement and evidence-based practice, and (14) lifelong learning.

Comprehensive care

Family medicine in the EMR takes a holistic approach, addressing not only physical health but also psychological, social, and environmental factors.[22] This comprehensive model reflects one of the core values of primary healthcare, which is widely embraced across the region.[23]

FPs strive to provide care that supports the whole person, encompassing all dimensions of health and wellbeing. However, in some settings, their role within primary healthcare centres may be more focused, concentrating on areas such as non-communicable diseases, childcare, or women's health. Notably, mental health services are offered by only a small proportion of FPs in the region.[17]

Continuity of care

Fostering a continuous therapeutic relationship between physicians and patients is a cornerstone of the family medicine specialty in the EMR. Patients in Oman, for example, have expressed appreciation for interpersonal continuity at the primary care level.[24] However, the level of continuity of care was found to be low in countries with high population mobility such as Saudi Arabia.[25] Saudi Arabia is undergoing a transformative journey through its Vision 2030 initiative, aiming to achieve 'a FP for every family' while integrating advanced technologies, such as electronic health records, to enhance continuity of care.[26]

Patient-centred care

Patient-centred care is recognized as a fundamental value of family medicine in the EMR. While there is significant interest in promoting shared decision-making and patient-centred care in the region, several challenges have been identified.[27,28] These include time constraints, increased costs, limited healthcare resources, some physicians' tendency to dominate decisions, and patients' preference for deferring to their doctors.[27,28] Cultural and religious factors also influence these dynamics.[28] Notably, in Sudan, the orientation toward patient-centred care remained limited even after family medicine training.[29]

Compassionate care

The countries of the EMR are deeply rooted in religious and paternalistic cultural values, which often shape behaviour and interactions.[30] FPs in this region are not only influenced by these values but also embody them in their relationships with patients. Compassion and humanism are hallmarks of their approach to care, reflecting a genuine willingness to assist others and exemplifying the essence of medicine in their daily interactions.

Equity and access

Achieving equity and ensuring access to care lie at the heart of universal health coverage, a goal the region is steadfastly striving to realise. The family practice–based model of care has been identified as a key pathway to advancing universal health coverage within the EMR.[11] FPs in primary healthcare centres play a pivotal role in facilitating timely access to essential healthcare services for all community members, with a particular focus on underserved and marginalized populations. Notably, family physician–led initiatives have been implemented in EMR countries such as Lebanon to address the needs of refugees and internally displaced persons, further underscoring their critical contributions to health equity. Yet challenges in equitable access to healthcare remain a reality in the region.[12,13]

Prevention and health promotion

FPs in the EMR play a crucial role in preventive care, engaging in activities such as vaccination, health screenings, lifestyle counselling, and the early detection of non-communicable diseases. These efforts are consistently observed across nearly all countries in the region. In Qatar, for example, the introduction of a family medicine–based model within primary healthcare has been particularly impactful, successfully shifting the focus from curative to preventive care.[31,32]

Cultural sensitivity and respect for diversity

Cultural sensitivity is a cornerstone of family medicine, especially in the culturally and ethnically diverse EMR. FPs are trained to recognize and respect the cultural, religious, and social factors that shape patients' health and influence their healthcare decisions. This approach is particularly vital in countries like Lebanon and the United Arab Emirates, where diverse ethnic communities coexist, emphasizing the importance of culturally adapted care.

Community-oriented care

Family medicine in the EMR places a strong focus on community health, with practitioners actively participating in health education, community health programmes, and public health initiatives. Training in community health has been a foundational element of the Arab Board certification in family medicine.[22]

Family medicine trainees are equipped with the skills to assess the health needs of their communities and implement effective interventions in collaboration with community leaders and stakeholders. A noteworthy example is Jordan's adoption of the family health team approach, which integrates family medicine into the public health system while prioritizing community-based care.[20] In Kuwait, FPs working in primary healthcare centres implement interventions based on the needs and priorities of the community.[13]

Advocacy

Although family medicine was introduced in the EMR more than four decades ago, raising awareness about the discipline remains a significant challenge. This lack of awareness is evident among the public, medical students, and even healthcare professionals from other specialties. While the role of FPs in managing chronic conditions and promoting prevention is generally viewed positively, familiarity with the specialty itself or direct encounters with family medicine remain limited.[33]

FPs in the region have consistently recognized the need to advocate for their specialty, clarifying their role and contributions to healthcare. Advocacy has become a core mission for most family medicine scientific societies and associations in the EMR, which leverage traditional media and social media platforms to raise awareness and highlight the value of family medicine.

Resilience and adaptability

In a region where nearly half of the countries are impacted by conflict, resilience and adaptability are essential values in family medicine. These qualities enable FPs and family medicine–based care models to effectively address challenges such as conflict, displacement, and resource limitations. For instance, FPs in Lebanon, Syria, and Palestine have demonstrated remarkable ingenuity in delivering high-quality care despite constrained resources. In Lebanon, FPs have taken the lead in mobile health clinics, providing essential healthcare services to displaced and underserved populations.

This adaptability and resilience are further exemplified on a broader scale across the region, where primary care physicians, including FPs, were at the forefront of the COVID-19 pandemic response.[34] They adapted to rapidly changing circumstances and embraced new norms, reaffirming their critical role in ensuring uninterrupted and effective care delivery.

Collaboration and teamwork

Various models of family practice are employed across the region, including the single-clinician model and the multidisciplinary family medicine–based approach. The single-clinician model is predominantly observed in private solo practices of FPs. In contrast, the team-based approach, characterized by collaboration with healthcare professionals such as nurses, social workers, midwives, and other specialists, is more commonly implemented in primary healthcare centres and ambulatory facilities, whether in public or private settings.

FPs also collaborate with other sectors, such as education and social services, to address social determinants of health, reflecting the holistic nature of their practice. Furthermore, the relationships between FPs and specialists are generally positive, fostering a collaborative environment that benefits patient care.[35]

Ethical practice and professionalism

Ethical principles such as maintaining patient confidentiality, obtaining informed consent, ensuring fairness in care, transparency, accountability, and respecting patient autonomy are fundamental values in family medicine throughout the EMR. These principles are consistently upheld, reflecting a commitment to professional integrity and ethical standards in interactions with patients, families, and other healthcare providers.

Professionalism is deeply embedded in family medicine practice and is a cornerstone of training programmes in the region, ensuring that FPs uphold these values in every aspect of their work.

Quality improvement and evidence-based practice

The core values of family medicine in the EMR emphasize 'patient first' and 'patient safety' as essential principles, with a strong emphasis on evidence-based care to ensure that services meet global healthcare standards.

Many countries in the region are prioritizing the enhancement of care quality through evidence-based practices. This includes integrating the latest research and clinical guidelines into practice, alongside a commitment to ongoing professional development. However, patient and family engagement in patient safety faces several challenges, including a lack of awareness about the role patients play in preventing harm, cultural barriers, absence of relevant policies, and sometimes negative attitudes from healthcare providers toward active patient involvement.[36]

Lifelong learning

Family medicine in the EMR is marked by a strong commitment to both personal and professional development, with a focus on engaging in learning activities that ultimately improve patient outcomes. Nearly all scientific societies and associations for family medicine organize regular conferences aimed at enhancing the knowledge and skills of practicing FPs.

In some countries in the EMR such as Lebanon, Bahrain, and United Arab Emirates, earning continuous medical education points is mandatory; many other institutions or universities in the region require this for academic FPs as well. However, the absence of specific regulations in some countries may limit physicians' participation in such activities.[37]

Despite these challenges, FPs in the region are generally highly motivated to pursue continuous professional development. Many are also working towards additional diplomas or university degrees, which further strengthen their expertise and enhance their ability to provide high-quality care.[35]

IMPLICATIONS AND APPLICATIONS

The core values of family medicine in the EMR share many similarities, though they also reflect differences influenced by cultural, political, and economic conditions; traditions; and healthcare contexts. However, there is a notable lack of research defining and exploring the practice of family medicine core values in the region, and no unified statement has been published on these values. This work aims to lay the groundwork for such a statement.

FPs in the region are introduced to these core values during their training in various family medicine programmes. Graduates of these programmes strive to implement these values, yet they often face unique limitations within their respective contexts that hinder or prevent full implementation.

The primary challenge in the region is the limited access to family medicine, primarily due to the low number of available FPs. The WHO, in collaboration with several stakeholders, is making significant efforts to strengthen family medicine in the region.[19] The most recent initiative is the launch of the regional professional diploma in family medicine in partnership with the Arab Board of Health Specializations, WONCA EMR, and various United Nations agencies.[18,38] This diploma, along with other initiatives, will help produce physicians trained in family medicine who are equipped to implement the discipline's core values. It is also crucial to emphasize the need for exposure to family medicine in undergraduate medical education across the region, as this would help spark greater interest in the specialty among future doctors.[33] This is already available in certain undergraduate medical education programmes, but more stress should be on teaching medical students the family medicine core values.

Simultaneously, national policies that support family practice (or family medicine–oriented primary care) as the central entry point into healthcare systems in many regional countries must be developed and strengthened. Such policies would improve access to quality healthcare and contribute to achieving universal health coverage. Several countries in the region have already embarked on improving access to care and integrating family medicine–based models which emphasize person-centred care. For these efforts to succeed, family medicine values must be embedded within these interventions. Offering integrated healthcare services based on family medicine will facilitate the implementation of key values such as comprehensive care, continuity of care, and patient-centred care. Strengthening health systems, including the introduction of technologies such as electronic health records, registries, and telemedicine, will also be essential to supporting the integration of these values in clinical practice.

Raising awareness of family medicine among the public and healthcare providers in the region is another critical necessity.[33] Highlighting the core values and principles of family medicine offers an excellent opportunity to educate both the public and healthcare professionals about what FPs do and how they can offer distinct approaches to care. This can be achieved through innovative interventions, including the use of social media and influencers. Additionally, emphasizing the vital role FPs play within multidisciplinary teams and fostering collaborative relationships with other healthcare providers can help portray a more accurate and positive image of family medicine.

Scientific societies and associations that are currently members in WONCA EMR, and those that will join in the future, should continue to organize continuous professional development activities for their members. These efforts will improve the quality of care provided and increase awareness of family medicine's core values. Including topics related to these values in conferences will also promote discussion and experience-sharing across different countries.

It is essential for countries in the EMR to collaborate on regional training programmes and knowledge-sharing platforms that align with shared values while respecting cultural diversity. Developing a dynamic monitoring framework at the regional level to assess how well these shared values are integrated into actions would be a valuable step forward. Such a framework could guide the development of family medicine by mapping shared values and context-specific actions across the region.

CONCLUSION

The core values of family medicine in the EMR embody a commitment to addressing diverse healthcare challenges while honouring the region's unique cultural, social, and economic contexts. These values serve as foundational principles, guiding FPs and healthcare systems in delivering high-quality, equitable, and sustainable care. It is crucial for these values and principles to inform key actions, including training, policy development, and patient engagement.

The future of family medicine in the EMR hinges on its capacity to harmonize shared aspirations with local realities. By integrating values, principles, vision, mission, and context-specific competencies, the region can foster a cohesive and resilient primary care system. This approach not only strengthens the discipline of family medicine but also enables it to effectively address the unique and evolving health needs of the EMR's diverse populations.

REFERENCES

1. Brennan R, Hajjeh R, Al-Mandhari A. Responding to health emergencies in the Eastern Mediterranean region in times of conflict. *Lancet* 2022;399:e20–2. https://doi.org/10.1016/S0140-6736(20)30069-6
2. Girgis L, Van Gurp G, Zakus D, Andermann A. Physician experiences and barriers to addressing the social determinants of health in the Eastern Mediterranean region: A qualitative research study. *BMC Health Serv Res* 2018;18(1):614. https://doi.org/10.1186/s12913-018-3408-z
3. WONCA. Strong Family Practice and Universal Health Coverage in the Middle East, 2014 [Available from: https://www.globalfamilydoctor.com/News/StrongfamilypracticeanduniversalhealthcoverageintheMiddleEa.aspx]

4. Pettersson T, Högbladh S, Öberg M. Organized violence, 1989–2018 and peace agreements. *J Peace Res* 2019;56:589–603.

5. WONCA. Family Medicine in the Eastern Mediterranean Region [Available from: https://www.globalfamilydoctor.com/AboutWonca/PresidentsBlog/FamilyMedicineintheEasternMediterraneanRegion.aspx]

6. WONCA. Region: East Mediterranean [Available from: https://www.globalfamilydoctor.com/AboutWonca/Regions/EastMediterranean2.aspx accessed 28 Dec 2024]

7. WONCA. Member Organizations: East Mediterranean Region [Available from: https://www.globalfamilydoctor.com/AboutWonca/Regions/East%20MediterraneanMemberOrganizations.aspx]

8. World Bank. World Bank Country Classifications by Income Level for 2024–2025. [Available from: https://blogs.worldbank.org/en/opendata/world-bank-country-classifications-by-income-level-for-2024-2025]

9. Worldmeter. Countries in the World by Population, 2024 [Available from: https://www.worldometers.info/world-population/population-by-country/]

10. Health and Well-being Profile of the Eastern Mediterranean Region: An Overview of the Health Situation in the Region and Its Countries in 2019. Cairo: WHO Regional Office for the Eastern Mediterranean, 2020.

11. Salah H, Kidd M, eds. Family Practice in the Eastern Mediterranean Region: Primary Health Care for Universal Health Coverage. 1st ed. CRC Press 2019. https://doi.org/10.1201/9780429298295

12. van Weel C, Alnasir F, Farahat T, et al. Primary healthcare policy implementation in the Eastern Mediterranean region: Experiences of six countries. *Eur J Gen Pract* 2018;24:39–44. https://doi.org/10.1080/13814788.2017.1397624

13. Nashat N, Hadjij R, Al Dabbagh AM, et al. Primary care healthcare policy implementation in the Eastern Mediterranean region: Experiences of six countries: Part II. *Eur J Gen Pract* 2020;26:1–6. https://doi.org/10.1080/13814788.2019.1640210

14. World Health Organization – Regional Office for the Eastern Mediterranean. Intercountry Consultation on Family Practice in the Eastern Mediterranean Region, 2007 [Available from: http://applications.emro.who.int/docs/WHO_EM_HCD_083_E_en.PDF]

15. Arya N, Gibson C, Ponka D, et al. Family medicine around the world: Overview by region: The Besrour papers – a series on the state of family medicine in the world. *Can Fam Physician* 2017;63(6):436–41.

16. Al Nasir FA. Challenges facing family medicine in the EMRO region. Annual Congress & Medicare Expo on Primary Healthcare, 2016 [Available from: https://www.iomcworld.org/proceedings/challenges-facing-family-medicine-in-the-emro-region-48641.html]

17. Osman H, Romani M, Hlais S. Family medicine in Arab countries. *Fam Med* 2011;43:37–42.

18. Salah H, Mataria A, Wajid G, et al. Promoting family practice-based model of care: The role of WHO's professional diploma in family medicine in the Eastern Mediterranean region. *East Mediterr Health J* 2021;27(8):743–4. https://doi.org/10.26719/2021.27.8.743

19. World Health Organization. Scaling up family practice: Progressing toward universal health coverage. WHO EMRO Regional Committee Resolution EM/RC63/R2. WHO EMRO: Cairo, 2016 [Available from: http://applications.emro.who.int/docs/RC63_Resolutions_2016_R2_19197_EN.pdf?ua=]

20. Khader Y, Al Nsour M, Abu Khudair S, et al. Strengthening primary healthcare in Jordan for achieving universal health coverage: A need for family health team approach. *Healthcare* 2023;11:2993. https://doi.org/10.3390/healthcare11222993

21. Soliman SSA, Hopayian K. Egypt: On the brink of universal family medicine. *Br J Gen Pract* 2019;69:82. https://doi.org/10.3399/bjgp19X701069

22. Arab Board of Health Specializations. Training Guide [Available from: https://www.arab-board.org/Specialties/Family-Medicine]

23. Eastern Mediterranean Public Health Network (EMPHNET). Strengthening Primary Healthcare through the Family Health Team Approach, 2024 [Available from: https://emphnet.net/media/4e2p0nyw/strengthening-primary-healthcare-a-summary-of-emphnet-roadmap.pdf]

24. Al-Azri M, Ganguly SS. Patients' views of interpersonal continuity of care in four primary health care centres of urban Oman. *Sultan Qaboos Univ Med J* 2009;9(3):287–95.

25. Almalki ZS, Alahmari AK, Alajlan SA, et al. Continuity of care in primary healthcare settings among patients with chronic diseases in Saudi Arabia. *SAGE Open Med* 2023;11:20503121231208648. https://doi.org/10.1177/20503121231208648

26. Alshammari SA. Preparedness to implement 'a family physician for every family,' which is the magic recipe for cost-effective health care for all: Viewpoint. *J Nat Sci Med* 2023;6:95–100. https://doi.org/10.4103/jnsm.jnsm_141_22

27. Alsulamy N, Lee A, Thokala P, et al. Views of stakeholders on factors influencing shared decision-making in the Eastern Mediterranean region: A systematic review. *East Mediterr Health J* 2021;27(3):300–11. https://doi.org/10.26719/emhj.20.139

28. Rawaf S, Alnasir F, Saad NE. Barriers, challenges, and way forward for implementation of person-centred care model of patient and physician consultation: A survey of patients' perspective from Eastern Mediterranean countries. *Middle East J Fam Med* 2015;13(3):4–11. https://doi.org/10.5742/mewfm.2015.92672

29. Khalid Ghaffer M, Hunskaar S, Abdelrahman SH, et al. Impact on core values of family medicine from a 2-year master's programme in Gezira, Sudan: Observational study. *BMC Fam Pract* 2019;20:145. https://doi.org/10.1186/s12875-019-1037-1

30. Yousuf AAAA, Stewart DC, Kane T, et al. Health professionals' views and experiences of breaking bad news in the Eastern Mediterranean region: A scoping review. *Front Med* 2024;11:1440867. https://doi.org/10.3389/fmed.2024.1440867

31. Syed MA, Al Mujalli H, Kiely CM, et al. Development of a model to deliver primary health care in Qatar. *Integr Healthc J* 2020;2:e000040. https://doi.org/10.1136/ihj-2020-000040

32. PHCC's Family Medicine Model Effective in Delivering Holistic Primary Care [Available from: https://thepeninsulaqatar.com/article/21/08/2022/phccs-family-medicine-model-effective-in-delivering-holistic-primary-care]

33. Maraqa B, Nazzal Z, Zink T. A systematic review of Arab community perceptions and awareness of family medicine. *BJGP Open* 2024. https://doi.org/10.3399/BJGPO.2024.0104

34. Qidwai W, et al. Primary health care in pandemics: Barriers, challenges, and opportunities. *World Fam Med* 2021;19:6–11. https://doi.org/10.5742/MEWFM.2021.94090

35. Helou M, Rizk GA. State of family medicine practice in Lebanon. *J Fam Med Prim Care* 2016;5(1):51–5. https://doi.org/10.4103/2249-4863.184623

36. Abdi Z, Ravaghi H, Sarkhosh S, et al. Patient and family engagement in patient safety in the Eastern Mediterranean region: A scoping review. *BMC Health Serv Res* 2024;24:765. https://doi.org/10.1186/s12913-024-11198-3

37. Younes NA, AbuAlRub R, Alshraideh H, et al. Engagement of Jordanian physicians in continuous professional development: Current practices, motivation, and barriers. *Int J Gen Med* 2019;12:475–83. https://doi.org/10.2147/IJGM.S232248

38. World Health Organization. Regional Professional Diploma in Family Medicine. [Available from: https://www.emro.who.int/uhc-health-systems/access-health-services/family-medicine.html]

CHAPTER 6

General practice/family medicine core values in the European region

Katharina Schmalstieg-Bahr,
Helen Alter, Nina Monteiro,
Nena Kopcavar Gucek,
and Dorien Zwart

REGIONAL DESCRIPTION

The region covered by WONCA Europe is extensive and includes countries that geographically might be considered to be East Mediterranean, transcontinental, or Asia. The region extends all the way from Greenland (adjacent to northeastern Canada) to the eastern tip of Russia (in close proximity to Alaska in the United States just across the Bering Sea). Europe includes the islands of Iceland and Ireland bordering on the Atlantic Ocean; the United Kingdom separated from Continental Europe by the North Sea; the Nordic countries to the north and others around the Baltic Sea (e.g. Estonia, Latvia); Germany, Austria, and other countries in central Europe; those along the north Mediterranean such as Portugal and Italy; countries located around the Black (e.g. Romania, Türkiye) and Caspian (e.g. Georgia, Azerbaijan) Seas, through to the 'stans' (e.g. Turkmenistan, Kyrgyzstan) – Central Asian nations formerly part of the Soviet Republic. WONCA includes Israel in the European region, although it is located in the east Mediterranean. The Russian Federation (Russia) covers an area of about 17 million square kilometres, making it by far the largest country in the world, but much of it is relatively under-populated, with most people living in the western region around Moscow (Figure 6.1).

DOI: 10.1201/9781003542353-6

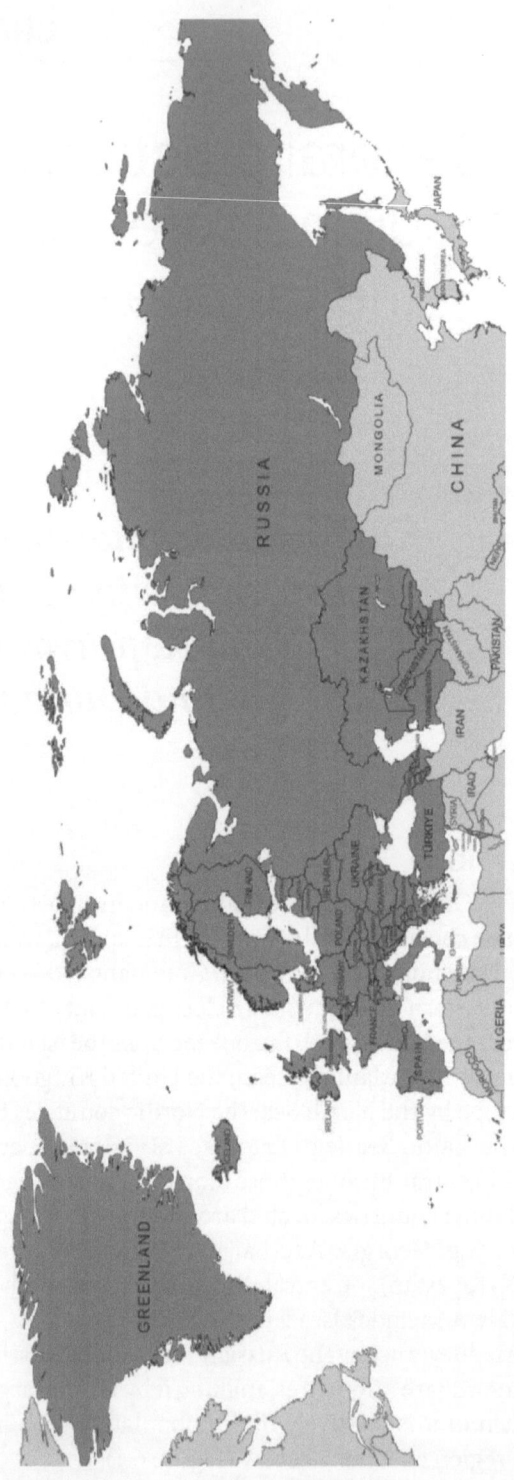

FIGURE 6.1 Map of Europe.

Source: Created using mapchart.net

Countries in WONCA Europe range from Russia, with its vast land mass and a population nearing 144 million, to tiny micro-states such as Liechtenstein and Monaco, with populations around 40,000. Of these 53 WONCA-designated European areas (which excludes the Vatican City, although it is officially a sovereign state), the majority (33) are high-income countries (HIC). However, there are also 14 upper-middle-income (e.g. Romania, Serbia) and five lower-middle-income countries such as Ukraine and Tajikistan. There is also diversity in life expectancy, with Turkmenistan at 68.2 years, whereas the average life expectancy of people in HICs is generally more than 80 years, topped by Monaco at 86.6 years.

There are many cultures in Europe and 24 official languages, with more than 200 other languages spoken across the continent.[1] The region is home to many religions, including Christianity, Islam, and Judaism, as well as indigenous spiritual practices. The main Christian divisions are Roman Catholicism in the west and southwest (e.g. Italy, Spain, Poland), Protestantism (northern countries), and Eastern Orthodoxy (in the east and southeast, especially Greece, Russia, and Serbia). Islam is the second-largest religion, with the majority of Muslim communities in western Europe resulting from immigration, as well as centuries-old Muslim communities in the Baltic region.

WONCA Europe (WE) became of one the seven WONCA world regional branches in 1995. It represents 47 member organizations from 43 of the 53 WONCA-designated European countries and more than 90,000 family doctors in the European region. There are nine WE special interest groups and six networks, each with a different focus in order to promote and support 'professional development, research, education and quality improvement'.[2]

These 43 countries depict a broad spectrum of cultural and socioeconomic characteristics, and each country has its own healthcare system, which shapes the setting in which family doctors work. Despite the existence of a European definition of general practice/family medicine and common core values,[3] the daily work of family doctors within the European region varies tremendously.

For instance, in some countries, family doctors function as gatekeepers, for example, in the Netherlands, Norway, and Denmark and within the Portuguese public healthcare system (excluding the private health sector). In other countries, such as Austria, Germany, the Czech Republic, and Greece, there is no gatekeeping system,[4] which means that patients are not required to have a family doctor and/or may consult any doctor of any specialty without contacting their family doctor first. This will influence how family doctors perceive their role within the healthcare system and how they implement family medicine core values such patient-centred care.[5]

There are also significant differences regarding the training of family doctors and their scope of practice. For example, in some countries family doctors deliver women health services, such as in Portugal and Denmark, where family

doctors offer care regarding family planning/contraception, prenatal, and pae-
diatric care, whereas in Spain they do not. This may also lead to differences
among European family doctors' daily work, such as continuity or cooperation
in care. Nevertheless, the debate and dialogue about common family medicine
core values and principles with the European region have been going on for
over decades.

Development of WONCA Europe core values and principles

Long before WE was founded, the debate about family medicine core values
started to be decentralised in individual countries. Over 60 years ago Dutch
family doctors formulated three core values (continuity of care, generalism,
person-centredness). These were reconfirmed in 2019 after a nationwide discussion among hundreds of family doctors, and a fourth value (cooperation)
was added.[6] In late 1990s, English family doctors saw gatekeeping, commissioning, and managed care as core values,[7] and in 2001 the Norwegian College
of General Practice launched their statement identifying the seven theses that
characterize the principles, purposes, and core values of general practice,[8]
which led to the seven joint core values published by the Nordic Federation
of General Practice[9] (see Chapter 2). As described in that chapter, in 2023 WE
published its core values and principles, which are similar to the Nordic ones
(person-centred, equity of, continuity of, science-oriented, professionalism
in, cooperation in, and community-orientated care).[3]

Originally produced by the Swiss College of Primary Care in 2005 and later
revised in 2011 and 2023, the WONCA 'tree' accompanies the *WE Core Values
and Principles*. It depicts the interrelationship of core competencies, essential
application features, and the implementation that characterizes the discipline
and underlines the complexity of the family medicine specialty. Around the
base of the tree is written 'One Health, Planetary Health and Sustainability is
the bedrock of General Practice/Family Medicine' (Figure 6.2).

Processes

From our personal knowledge and examination of member organizations'
websites, and from talking with colleagues at former WONCA Europe conferences and special interest meetings including the European Association
for Quality and Patient Safety in General Practice/Family Medicine (EQuiP)
since 2007, we have identified that there are considerable differences regarding the distribution, implementation, and use of the *WE Core Values and
Principles* among the 43 European countries. The German Society of General
Practice and Primary Care, for example, has used the same wording, such
as patient-centred care or continuity of care, for many years when describ-
ing the goals and gist of the specialty but without explicitly defining them

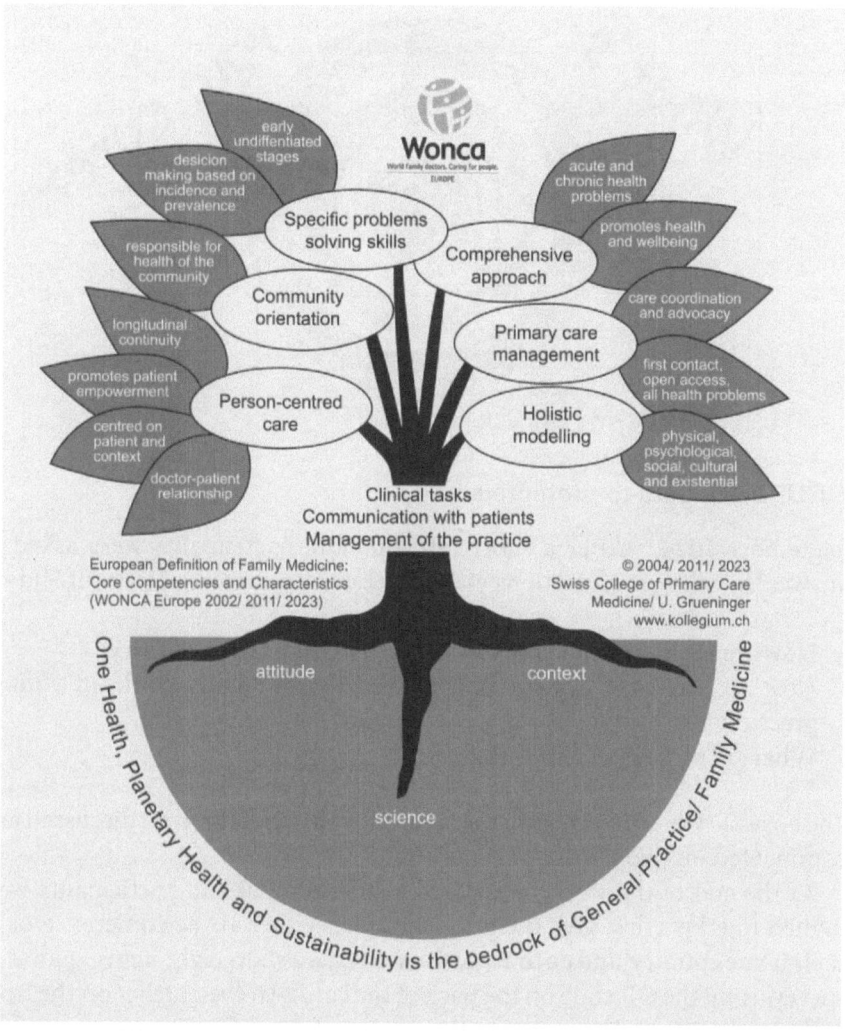

Figure 6.2 The WONCA Europe tree.

as core values. They only added the *WE Core Values and Principles* to their homepage in 2024. In contrast, the Netherlands, which borders Germany, had already defined core values very early, and professional organizations such as the Dutch College of GPs and the Dutch Association of GPs have built these as fundamentals into their policies, guidelines, quality of care policy, and educational programmes.

To further explore to what extent the *WE Core Values and Principles* are known to European family doctors and how they influence their daily work, we held a workshop during the WONCA Europe conference in Dublin in

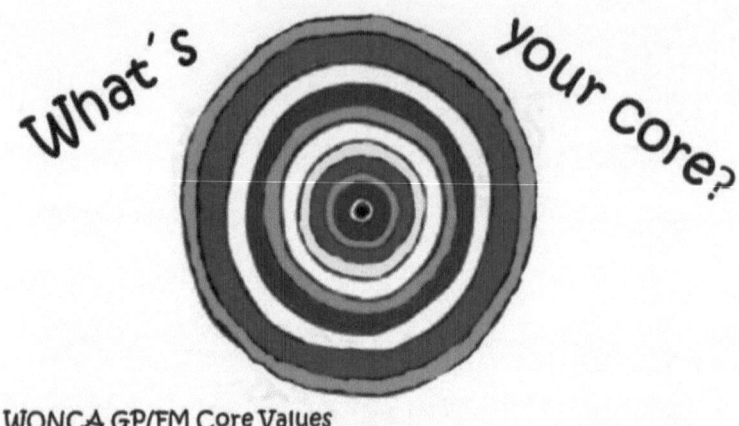

WONCA GP/FM Core Values

FIGURE 6.3 Card to promote survey.

September 2024.[10] After a short introduction, participants were asked to answer the following questions via the online-based poling platform Slido:

- How are the European core values recognised in your country?
- How are the core values implemented in your daily work, in your practice?
- What are obstacles or facilitators?

The answers were projected on the screen for participants, who discussed and commented on them.

At the end of the workshop, cards were given out and participants were invited to take a few, give them to colleagues either at the conference or in their home country, and encourage them to take a short eight-item explorative survey using the QR code on the back of the card. An eye-catcher on the front of the card presented tree rings in the colours of many European country flags to encourage looking inside the WONCA 'tree' (Figure 6.3).

Findings

Workshop findings
The results of the workshop poll showed a broad range regarding the publicity from 'very recognised'/'well recognised' to 'moderately' to 'not yet recognised/unknown'. If the core values were known, they were implemented in 'GP education and research' or 'practice and study'. Participants stated that core values were implemented in their own daily work in terms of 'patient-centredness', 'equality', 'continuity', 'cooperation', 'teamwork', and 'practice management'.

Some kept the core values 'deeply inside' or 'in the back of [their] head', while others admitted that 'it's a fight' and 'we try'; some were especially 'fighting the system for equity' or found it difficult 'due to external drivers'. 'Time', 'money', and 'bureaucracy/administrative rules' were identified as the biggest obstacles. This included aspects such as 'floods of information to stay on top of', the 'funding of the primary care system', or the need for 'more GPs for continuity of care'. Furthermore, 'patient expectations' were also mentioned as an obstacle.

Survey results

One hundred and fifty family doctors from over 10 countries answered the survey, many from either Estonia ($n = 34$) or Slovenia ($n = 28$). Nine were still GP trainees, seven academics, and four had a different working position, such as retired or manager. Most of the participants had practised for more than 20 years. The majority stated that the *WE Core Values and Principles* were helpful for clinicians in their daily work (Figure 6.4), but identified lack of control, time constraints due to GP deficiency, and too much bureaucracy but also unfamiliarity with the core values as implementation barriers.

Survey participants suggested better practice organization/management and teamwork and more knowledge and training as facilitators for

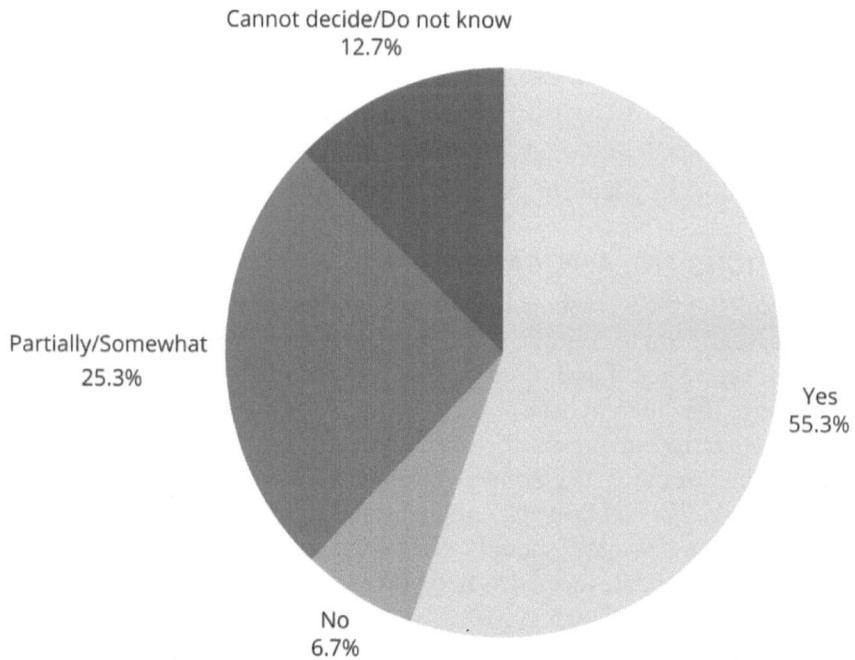

FIGURE 6.4 Is the European statement on core values helpful for clinicians in their daily work?

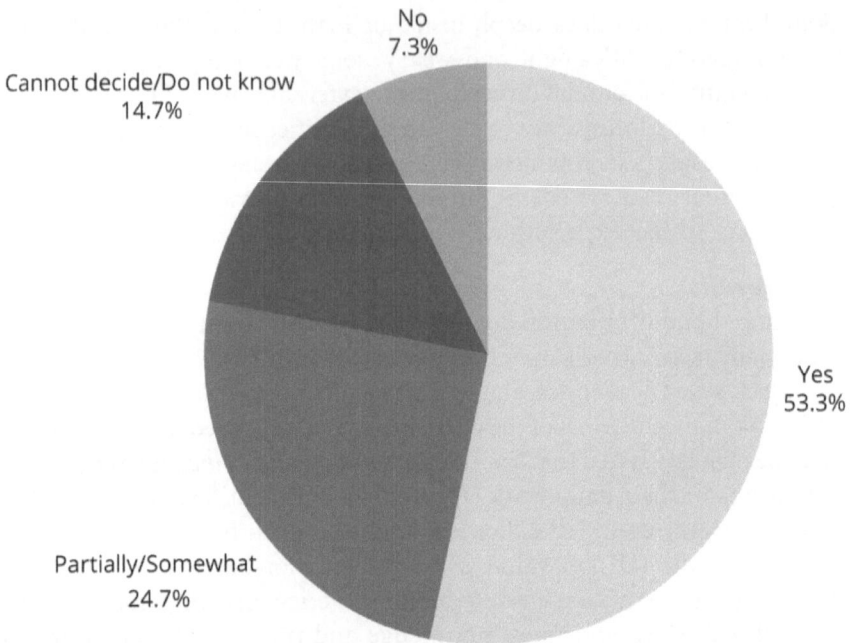

No
7.3%

Cannot decide/Do not know
14.7%

Yes
53.3%

Partially/Somewhat
24.7%

FIGURE 6.5 Are these core values taken into consideration when planning undergraduate and postgraduate curricula in your institution/environment?

implementation of core values in the daily clinical routine. The *WE Core Values and Principles* were taken into consideration most often during the planning of undergraduate or postgraduate curricula (Figure 6.5).

IMPLICATIONS AND APPLICATIONS

As the results of the workshop and the survey show, much work needs to be done to actually implement the *WE Core Values and Principles* in all 43 WE countries. The degree of utilisation in daily practice will probably vary to some extent due to the different healthcare systems. Nevertheless, efforts should be made to help European family doctors work according to the *WE Core Values and Principles* as much as possible. Within the Global Core Values project, the *WE Core Values and Principles* might be an inspiration for other WONCA regions and vice versa: WE should reflect upon core values from other parts of the world and update its own as necessary.

ACKNOWLEDGMENT

The authors would like to acknowledge Roar Maagaard for his help and intellectual input.

REFERENCES

1. Tomedes. European Languages: Exploring the Languages of Europe, 2024 [Available from: https://www.tomedes.com/translator-hub/european-languages accessed Jan 2025]
2. Toplek B. The WONCA Europe Secretariat, 2025 [Available from: https://www.globalfamilydoctor.com/AboutWonca/Regions/Europe.aspx accessed Jan 2025]
3. WONCA Europe. The European Definition of General Practice/Family Medicine, 2002:35.
4. Union OE. Health at a glance: Europe 2016. State of Health in the EU Cycle Paris: OECD Publishing, 2016 [Available from: https://www.oecd.org/en/publications/health-at-a-glance-europe-2016_9789264265592-en.html]
5. Schmalstieg-Bahr K, Popert K, Scherer M. The role of general practice in complex health care system. *Fron Med* 2021;8:680695. https://doi.org/10.3389/fmed.2021.680695
6. van der Horst HE, de Wit N. Redefining the core values and tasks of GPs in the Netherlands (Woudschoten 2019). *Br J Gen Pract* 2020;70(690):38–9. https://doi.org/10.3399/bjgp20X707681
7. Dixon J, Holland P, Mays N. Primary care: Core values developing primary care: Gatekeeping, commissioning, and managed care. *Br Med J* 1998;317(7151):125–8. https://doi.org/10.1136/bmj.317.7151.125
8. Sigurdsson JA, Beich A, Stavdal A. A saga-in-progress: Challenges and milestones on our way toward the Nordic core values and principles of family medicine/general practice. *Front Med* 2021;8:681612. https://doi.org/10.3389/fmed.2021.681612
9. Nordic Federation of General Practice. Core values and principles of Nordic General Practice/Family Medicine. NFGP, 2020.
10. Zwart D, Alter H, Maagaard R, et al. Core values are the essentials of good quality GP/FM: How do we practice core values in Europe? 29th WONCA Europe Conference. Dublin, Ireland, 2024.

CHAPTER 7

Exploring core values in family/community medicine in Latin America

Jacqueline Ponzo,
Otto Hamann Echeverri,
Mónica Álvarez Jaramillo,
María Belén Giménez,
and Fabiano Gonçalves Guimarães

REGIONAL DESCRIPTION

The American continent is divided into three large regions: South America, Central America, and North America. The Caribbean Sea, which connects the three regions, is home to numerous islands, many of which are nation-states. Cultural criteria are commonly used in research and by international organizations to define regions. From this perspective, there are two large regions: firstly the English-speaking countries located in North America and the Caribbean and, secondly, the Spanish- or Portuguese-speaking countries located in South America, Central America, and the Caribbean. This latter region is what we recognize as Latin America.

The Latin American countries joined WONCA in 2004. Previously, from 1981 they were organized as the Ibero-American Confederation of Family Medicine (CIMF), together with Spain and Portugal, the two European countries from which they derive their languages. The Ibero-American region in WONCA has further consolidated in past two decades. It is organized into four subregions:

DOI: 10.1201/9781003542353-7

Mesoamerica (Cuba, Costa Rica, Mexico, Nicaragua, Panama, Puerto Rico, and the Dominican Republic), Andean countries (Bolivia, Colombia, Ecuador, Peru, and Venezuela), southern countries (Argentina, Brazil, Chile, Paraguay, and Uruguay), and Iberia (Spain and Portugal). For the purpose of this core values project, Spain and Portugal are included in Europe; hence, this chapter focuses on Latin America.

Our speciality goes by a variety of names within the region, including family medicine, general and family medicine, comprehensive general medicine, and family and community medicine. The name includes 'community' in Brazil, Costa Rica, Peru, the Dominican Republic, and Uruguay, and in some countries, such as Colombia, the training is in community-oriented specialists although the name remains family medicine. In 2019 the Executive Committee of CIMF resolved and later approved in 2021 for the name 'family medicine/family and community medicine' to be used in institutional documents. In this chapter we have abbreviated this to family medicine. All countries in the region that have a family medicine association are part of WONCA Iberoamericana – CIMF (one association per country). There are currently no family medicine associations in Honduras, Guatemala, or El Salvador.

All countries in Latin America are shown in Figure 7.1. The English-, French- or Dutch-speaking countries in Meso or Andrean America of Belize, Guyana, Suriname, and French Guiana do not have family medicine organizations and are not included in the Latin American region. French-speaking Haiti is included in the North American chapter.

A summary of sociodemographic and health coverage indicators in the countries of Latin America is presented in Table 7.1, regardless of whether they have family medicine member organizations in WONCA. The total population exceeds 630 million. Latin America covers an area of 20,038,800 km², with an average population density of 32 inhabitants/km². Fourteen per cent of the population is concentrated in the five most populous cities: Sao Paulo, Mexico City, Buenos Aires, Rio de Janeiro, and Bogota (with populations between 11 and 22 million).

There are extensive rural areas, particularly in mountains and jungles, often inhabited by indigenous peoples, often in conflict over territory claimed for resource exploitation by companies or governments. The percentage of the urban population is lowest in Guatemala, with 52%, and highest in Uruguay, with 95%.

The region's gross domestic product (GDP) per capita is 10,797 (US dollars at 2024 prices) with marked differences between countries, ranging from 2613 (Nicaragua) to 36,779 (Puerto Rico) or 22,798 (Uruguay), if Puerto Rico is excluded as an unincorporated territory of the United States.[1] Although the GDP of Latin America and the Caribbean grew in 2024, this is the lowest growth in the world since 2007: 1.9% compared to a global growth of 2.7% and

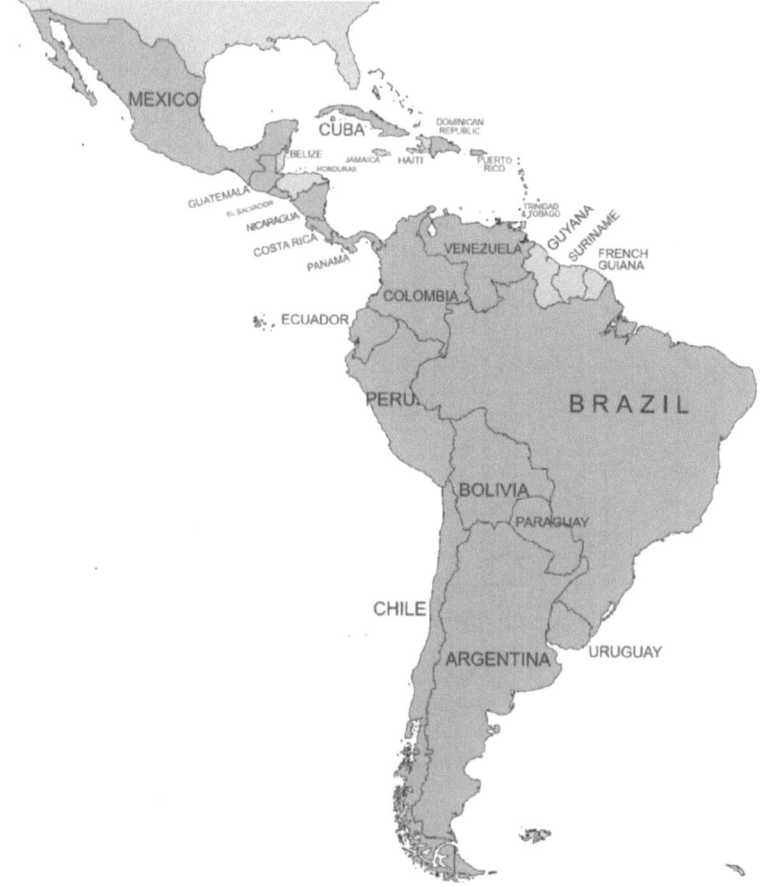

FIGURE 7.1 Map of countries in Latin America.

Source: mapchart.net

5.9% in the highest-income countries (see Table 7.2).[2] The World Bank categorizes most of the countries as upper-middle income, with Panama, Chile, and Uruguay being high income, and the poorest (lower-middle income) being Honduras, Nicaragua, and Bolivia.

Poverty and inequality are two serious problems that characterize the region. Although there was a reduction in poverty and extreme poverty at the regional level in 2024, poverty still affects 25% of the population, and extreme poverty affects 11% (70 million people). Less than USD 6.85 per day available to live on is the cut-off value for poverty and less than USD 2.15 dollars for extreme poverty. Thirty-one per cent of the population is considered vulnerable (at high risk of falling into poverty), with incomes ranging

TABLE 7.1 Sociodemographic and Health Characteristics of Latin American Countries

Country Name	Total Population in Millions	Life Expectancy at Birth	Population <15 Years	% Population <15 Years	% Urban Population	Fertility Rate (live births/woman)	Adolescent Fertility Rate (births/1000 women 15–19 years)	% Annual Population Growth Rate
Argentina	45.4	75.8	31.7	22.8	92.3	1.5	25.8	0.2
Bolivia	12.08	67.4	24.4	30.5	70.8	2.6	65.8	1.4
Brazil	210.30	74.9	33.5	20.2	87.6	1.6	42.9	0.4
Chile	19.55	79.2	35.5	17.8	87.9	1.3	7.7	0.5
Colombia	51.74	76.5	31.2	21.0	82.1	1.7	60.2	1.1
Costa Rica	5.08	79.3	33.5	19.8	82.0	1.3	26.5	0.4
Cuba	11.06	77.6	41.5	15.7	77.4	1.4	47.8	-0.4
Ecuador	17.82	76.6	28.0	25.5	64.6	1.9	57.0	0.9
El Salvador	6.28	72.0	26.5	25.6	74.8	1.8	54.9	0.5
Guatemala	17.84	71.2	22.2	32.7	52.7	2.3	69.1	1.5
Honduras	10.83	73.0	23.9	30.6	60.8	2.5	81.3	1.7
México	128.61	74.0	28.5	25.3	81.3	1.9	61.1	0.9
Nicaragua	6.73	74.5	24.9	29.6	59.6	2.2	94.1	1.4
Panamá	4.40	79.3	29.3	25.7	69.1	2.1	57.8	1.3
Paraguay	6.76	72.3	26.0	28.9	62.8	2.4	71.0	1.2
Perú	33.48	76.8	29.1	24.8	78.7	2.0	43.9	1.1
Puerto Rico	3.24	79.4	45.2	12.4	93.6	0.9	14.0	-0.1
Dominican Republic	11.23	74.2	27.3	27.2	83.8	2.3	53.6	0.9
Uruguay	3.39	76.5	35.5	19.1	95.7	1.4	26.5	-0.1
Venezuela	28.21	72.6	28.8	26.8	88.4	2.1	73.0	0.3

Source: Pan American Health Organization (PAHO), basic indicators, update 14.01.2025

between USD 6.85 and 14 per day[2]; hence more than half of the population (56%) is either in a state of vulnerability or poverty. In children, it is more dire. Poverty of children aged up to six years exceeds 50% in many countries. There are almost 100 million girls, boys, and adolescents up to the age of 17 years living in poverty, of whom 10 million are in extreme poverty.[3]

Inequality within each country is a serious problem, shown through the Gini index (Table 7.2). A value 0 corresponds to an egalitarian distribution, and 100 is the most unequal. The Gini index ranges from 38 (El Salvador) to 53.4 (Brazil). The median for the 17 countries with these data available is 46.[1] There is a shortage of jobs, which in the last decade had the lowest growth since 1950. Conversely, in 2021, there were an estimated 105 people whose wealth exceeded 1 billion dollars, together accumulating 3.6% of the wealth of the region.[4]

Although economic indicators look bleak, the regional wealth lies fundamentally in the natural and cultural diversity of each country, both closely linked to each other. Five countries are considered megadiverse, with 800 indigenous peoples, numbering 58 million (almost 10% of the total) and over 200 ancestral languages spoken in Brazil and more than 65 in Colombia.[5] The region extends from the vicinity of the South Pole to the south of the United States. Despite its cultural wealth, this population is largely marginalized from an economic and social point of view, and in many cases survival is threatened by the expansion of 'development' to its territories.[6]

The epidemiology of the region reflects this complex context. Chronic non-communicable diseases (NCDs) are highly prevalent, but so are numerous communicable diseases such as dengue, tuberculosis, HIV-AIDS, and others that are among the 'least attended to' diseases by health systems, such as Chagas disease or leprosy.[7]

Other prevalent health problems are those derived from poverty and violence. Gender violence is a serious public health problem in the region, with at least 11 women dying every day.[8] Brazil reported the highest number of femicides in Latin America in 2022, with 1463 cases. In the same year, Mexico registered 852, ranking second. With respect to rates, Honduras ranks first, with 7.2 cases per 100,000 women, followed by the Dominican Republic, with 2.4 cases per 100,000. In 2018, 14 of the 25 countries globally with the highest rates of femicide were in Latin America and the Caribbean. Since then there have been improvements, likely influenced by the social mobilisation of organized women. Homicides in general also constitute a public health problem linked to the presence of gangs, organized crime, and armed groups. The exposure of the younger population is especially serious. Adolescents in Latin America are five times more likely to die from homicide than their peers in the rest of the world.[9]

From a political point of view, internal conflict (including armed conflict), external interference, and authoritarianism, including state terrorism, have

TABLE 7.2 Main Economic Indicators of Latin American and Caribbean Countries

Country Name	GDP per Capita (USD)	Health Expenditure (% of GDP)	Out-of-Pocket Health Expenditure (% of total health expenditure)	Gini Index	Unemployment Rate (% of economically active population)
Argentina	14.18	9.1	28.0	42.9	9.8
Bolivia	3.69	6.3	30.5	47	4.8
Brazil	10.29	9.5	25.5	53.4	13.9
Chile	17.07	8.1	32.0	44.4	7.3
Colombia	6.945	7.2	23.0	50.4	11.2
Costa Rica	16.94	9.3	33.0	48.7	8.1
Cuba	9.61	11.7	10.0	N/A	2.5
Ecuador	6.61	7.5	27.0	45.7	5.2
El Salvador	5.39	6.8	40.0	38	6.5
Guatemala	5.76	5.6	54.0	48.3	2.8
Honduras	3.23	6.1	45.0	50.5	5.7
México	13.79	5.5	41.0	45.4	4.7
Nicaragua	2.61	5.0	42.0	46.2	6.2
Panamá	18.69	7.3	29.0	49.8	6.4
Paraguay	6.28	6.2	35.0	47.2	5.5
Perú	7.91	5.6	33.0	43.8	6.6
Puerto Rico	36.78	N/A	N/A	N/A	5.7
Dominican Republic	10.71	6.1	38.0	45.7	5.1
Uruguay	22.80	9.2	18.0	39.7	7.9
Venezuela	15.94	N/A	N/A	N/A	N/A

Notes: Per capita income figures are expressed in US dollars (USD) and correspond to the most recent year available.
Out-of-pocket health expenditure refers to the percentage of total health expenditure that is paid directly by individuals.
N/A: Data not available.
Source: Data retrieved 31 January 2025 from World Bank: https://data.worldbank.org/ and World Health Organization (WHO): https://www.who.int/data

ravaged the region in the last 50 years, constituting a constant threat to the stability of countries. However, there is democratic development, and the participation of the population through social movements is a characteristic of the region.

In this context, health systems that guarantee coverage with quality care to the entire population, and particularly to the most vulnerable people, are difficult to achieve, not only because of the scarce funds allocated to the sector but also because of the difficulty in coordinating human development processes.

Family medicine has had a progressive and uneven development in the region, in connection with universities and also through participation in health system reform processes such as the case of the Unified Health System in Brazil.[10] The number of family physicians in the region is insufficient but is increasing. In some countries, growth has been accelerated through the role of family medicine associations and their influence in the development of state policies and at the political level. For example, the number of family doctors in Brazil nearly doubled between 2019 and 2023, and the number of residency places in the Dominican Republic achieved a notable increase (Table 7.3).

The number of family physicians in the region is insufficient, and increasing this faces numerous challenges today. In addition to the low priority given to the specialty in many countries, there is also the low influx of candidates for residency positions in recent years.[11] In addition, there are the migratory movements of professionals and specialists who, having trained in our countries, then emigrate, particularly to Europe.

PROCESSES

The Core Values project was adopted in the region as an opportunity to strengthen the specialty and the WONCA Iberoamericana-CIMF organization to harmonize its implementation with processes already underway. The project was proposed in two stages: (1) the review of regional documents and (2) the collection of primary data through qualitative research interviewing family medicine specialists, leaders, and residents. This chapter presents the results of the first part of the project; the second part has not yet taken place.

WONCA Iberoamericana-CIMF has a history of more than 20 years of technical-political events called 'summits'. The first of these took place in Seville in 2002, and the most recent in Guatemala in 2022. The ninth Ibero-American Family Medicine Summit will take place in Montevideo, Uruguay, in May 2025. Each summit focuses on a topic of relevance for the region at that historical moment and highlights the importance of the specialty for the health of peoples. The summit process includes a period prior to the event in

TABLE 7.3 Number of Trained Family Physicians in Latin American Countries

Country	Number of doctors/10,000 Inhabitants**	Number of Trained Family Physicians*	Number of Family Physicians/10,000 Inhabitants	Number of Inhabitants/ Family Doctor
Argentina	51.1	6191	1.4	7335
Bolivia	12.8	800	0.7	15,097
Brazil	23.6	11,500	0.5	18,288
Chile	33.3	1498	0.8	13,053
Colombia	25.4	1300	0.3	39,798
Costa Rica	26.9	150	0.3	33,879
Cuba	95.4	32,517	29.4	340
Ecuador	23.1	2500	1.4	7130
El Salvador	16.2	200	0.3	31,402
México	25.9	29,350	2.3	4382
Nicaragua	6.8	90	0.1	74,786
Panamá	16.3	72	0.2	61,122
Paraguay	38.9	557	0.8	12,137
Perú	16.9	1300	0.4	25,750
Puerto Rico	29.3***	400	1.2	8103
Dominican Republic	24.3	2035	1.8	5519
Uruguay	46.7	650	1.9	5217
Venezuela	16.6	400	0.1	70,533

* Most updated data. Corresponds to years 2022 to 2024.

** Data taken from PAHO Basic Indicators.

*** Data not available in PAHO. Basic Indicators, calculated.

which technical documents are developed. From these, a summary document of each summit is produced, called the charter, followed by the name of the city hosting the event. In addition to the charters, there are the technical documents developed in the process and validated during the event in participatory workshops. In recent years, progress has been made in publishing these products. The charters and documents resulting from each summit constitute the main source of data for this stage of the project in Latin America (Table 7.4).

In addition to the summit documents, this review includes the CIMF website, its statutory documents, the description of the CIMF working groups, and the Proclamation for the Health of the Peoples. The development of the WONCA Iberoamericana residents and young doctors movement (Waynakay Movement) took place in the WONCA World Conference in Cancun, Mexico, in 2010. The proclamation was the result of the fourth Ibero-American Congress of Family Medicine that took place in Montevideo in March 2015 and produced a consensus document, as well as the installation of new working groups that were relevant in the following years to mark the identity of family medicine in the region.

FINDINGS

The efforts and orientations of the events and their documents reflect the values necessary for the practice of family medicine and the training of family physician specialists in Latin America.

As shown in Table 7.5, the values and principles for family medicine are articulated in the various charters:

1. Commitment to the person, the community, and equity.
2. Ethics and humanism.
3. Social and community responsibility.
4. Teaching vocation and continuous professional development.
5. Teamwork and collaboration.
6. Innovation and scientific development.
7. Quality in medical care.
8. Adaptability and resilience.

There is a focus on commitment and equity, as well as the quality of healthcare (care provided with humanism, respect, consideration of the diversity of people, and a rights perspective) and continuity of care. Family medicine is necessary for all people to access care. Participation is a value that runs through the practice of family medicine, required for the functioning of health teams and services, both through teamwork and community participation. Leadership is another aspect that repeatedly appears as a value or

TABLE 7.4 Summits and Derived Documents, CIMF, 2002–2022

Summit	Place	Date	Document	Motto
I	Seville, Spain	14–17 May 2002	Declaration of Seville	Committed to the health of the population
II	Santiago, Chile	5–6 October 2005	Santiago de Chile Commitment	The family doctor, a guarantee of quality and equity in the health systems of Latin America
III	Fortaleza, Brazil	29–30 April 2008	Charter of Fortaleza	Mission and challenges for family medicine and primary care in the 21st century: equity, integration, and quality in health systems
IV	Asunción, Paraguay	15–16 November 2011	Charter of Asunción	Family medicine and primary healthcare in renewed health: thought and action for the benefit of family health
V	Quito, Ecuador	11–12 April 2014	Charter of Quito	Universal coverage, family medicine, and social participation
VI	San José, Costa Rica	12–13 April 2016	Charter of San José	Universality, equity, and quality in health systems: family and community medicine as the axis
VII	Cali, Colombia	13–14 March 2018	Charter of Cali	Forty years of Alma Ata: family medicine and family health, a path to peace
VIII	Ciudad de Guatemala	10–11 November 2022	Charter of Guatemala	Family and community medicine, an essential specialty for the transformation of health systems in the 21st century

Source: WONCA Iberoamericana CIMF documents.

TABLE 7.5 Values and Principles of Family Medicine in Latin America From the Summit Charters

Seville Declaration 2002	Santiago, Chile Commitment 2005	Charter of Fortaleza 2008	Charter of Asunción 2011	Charter of Quito 2014	Charter of San José 2016	Charter of Cali 2018	Charter of Guatemala 2022
Commitment to the individual and the community	Commitment to equity and accessibility	Commitment to quality, equity, and comprehensiveness	Commitment to equity and the right to health	Commitment to universal coverage and equity	Commitment to universality and equity	Commitment to public health and equity	Commitment to equity, inclusiveness, and comprehensiveness
Ethics and humanism	Comprehensive and continuous care	Teaching vocation and continuing education	Comprehensive, continuous, and person-centred care	Comprehensive, continuous, and person-centred care	Ethics and social responsibility	Ethics and humanism	Ethics, rights perspective in health
Social responsibility	Ethics and social responsibility	Social responsibility and community commitment	Ethics and social responsibility	Ethics and social responsibility	Quality and humanism in care	Leadership and teamwork	Leadership for political advocacy and management
Teamwork and collaboration	Teamwork and collaboration	Ethics and humanism	Leadership and health management	Teaching vocation and continuing education	Teamwork and leadership	Teaching vocation and continuing education	Solidarity at different levels
Leadership and management in health	Teaching vocation and educational development	Scientific research and development	Teaching vocation and continuing education	Leadership and strengthening of the first level of care	Teaching vocation and continuing education	Scientific research and development	Participation: teamwork, openness to the community

(Continued)

TABLE 7.5 (Continued)

Seville Declaration 2002	Santiago, Chile Commitment 2005	Charter of Fortaleza 2008	Charter of Asunción 2011	Charter of Quito 2014	Charter of San José 2016	Charter of Cali 2018	Charter of Guatemala 2022
Teaching and educational vocation	Leadership in health management	Leadership and management in health	Scientific research and development	Scientific research and development	Commitment to research and innovation	Efficient management of health resources	Commitment to the diversity and context of the population
Commitment to equity and social justice	Commitment to research and innovation	Teamwork and collaboration	Quality in medical practice	Teamwork and interdisciplinary collaboration	Efficient management and sustainability	Commitment to mental health and wellbeing	Territorial perspective: integration of territorial processes in practice
Innovation and scientific development	Responsibility in the promotion of family medicine	Technological innovation and telemedicine	Teamwork and collaboration	Innovation and use of information technologies	Social participation and community empowerment	Social responsibility and community empowerment	Commitment to the biography of people, longitudinality
	Commitment to equity and accessibility	Commitment to vocational training	Adaptability and resilience				Culturally appropriate and respectful

attitude inherent to family medicine, within health teams, at a social level, at a political level for the improvement of health systems and services, and for the training of sufficient high-quality family physicians. The summits show a consistency over the years with respect to the commitment of family medicine to the health of the population, the quality of healthcare, and the transformation of health services in a way that guarantees equity.

There is a constant concern for professional quality, the training of family physicians with the appropriate skills, and increasing the number of training places. There is a commitment to the production of knowledge and research from and for primary healthcare and family medicine, guided by the problems of the population. There is also a commitment to the incorporation of technological developments, both in relation to medicine and in communication.

The sociodemographic profile of the region explains the sustained concern for equity. There is deep conviction of the power and capacity of family medicine to respond to needs. The aim is to transform health systems and services. It is not possible to advance the development of the family medicine specialty without achieving a place of relevance in health systems. Conversely, health systems will not be strong if they do not have family medicine. It is impossible to separate the training and development of the specialty from its overall role in the health system.

The territorial perspective is a feature that is gradually becoming consolidated. The integrated work with the environment, culture, and lifestyles of the population is expressed in different ways in the documents analyzed. This can be observed in the various territories of the region where family physicians work adapting to the needs and particularities of each place.

Other values can be identified by analyzing the profile of the working groups of WONCA Iberoamericana-CIMF. There are groups aimed at strengthening the specialty itself, such as the certification and recertification working group or the Ibero-American Confederation of Family Medicine research network. Other groups address the commitment to equity and inclusion: health and migration, sexual diversity and healthcare, and female family doctors, with a strong focus on prevention and care of situations of violence. Other groups are mainly oriented towards the incorporation of innovative perspectives in the specialty such as prevention from iatrogenic harm, planetary health, and community mental health.

The values and principles will be further explored during the second phase of the Core Values project in Latin America.

IMPLICATIONS AND APPLICATIONS

The Core Values project offers several opportunities to strengthen family medicine in the region. The opportunity to reflect on the values of family medicine at this time in the region is a great resource and a chance to stimulate the development of necessary innovations, as well as to strengthen the ethical perspective of our discipline. The definition of family medicine competencies is continually subject to review by our member associations and university settings, but an analysis of competencies based on values has not been carried out in the region. An analysis of this type could contribute to innovative planning of training based on values. The synthesis of core values that emerges from this project may also be a powerful resource for political advocacy that will continue to be necessary.

CONCLUSION

The speciality of family medicine is relatively young in Latin America. Its development is imbued with the complexity, diversity, and contradictions of the region, as well as its richness and cultural and territorial particularities. At the same time, family medicine is permeable to the health and social realities and the needs of the people, as well as to be strong and resilient in the search for the transformations that will make the right to access to healthcare possible. There needs to be an implicit integration of the population's health objectives with the development objectives of the specialty for this to happen. Professionalism in family medicine implies activism for health and for the improvement of health systems.

This commitment has been present in family medicine since its beginnings in the region and continues to this day. A specialist profile has been consolidated that is sensitive and integrated to reality, to the territories, to the people and committed to their continuous professional development, to the training of other specialists, to innovation, and to the production of knowledge through research.

REFERENCES

1. World Bank. World Bank Open Data, 2023 [Available from: https://data.worldbank.org accessed 1 Feb 2025]
2. Poverty and Equity Global Practice in the Latin America and Caribbean Region, World Bank Group, 2024 [Available from: https://documents1.worldbank.org/curated/en/099101724185031291/pdf/P50609514d5e250b919807109289007e31d.pdf accessed 1 Feb 2025]
3. Salmeron Gomez D, Engilbertsdottir S, Cuesta Leiva JA, et al. Global Trends in Child Monetary Poverty According to International Poverty Lines: World Bank; Washington, DC, 2023 [Available from: https://openknowledge.worldbank.org/handle/10986/40364 accessed 1 Feb 2025]
4. Economic Commission for Latin America and the Caribbean. Social Panorama of Latin America and the Caribbean 2023. Santiago: ECLAC, 2023:243 [Available from: https://www.cepal.org/es/publicaciones/68702-panorama-social-america-latina-caribe-2023-la-inclusion-laboral-como-eje-central accessed 1 Feb 2025]
5. Indigenous Peoples of Latin America and the Caribbean. UNESCO, 2023 [Available from: https://www.unesco.org/es/node/83544 accessed 1 Feb 2025]

6. Local and Indigenous Knowledge System (LINKS). UNESCO, 2023 [Available from: https://www.unesco.org/es/links/lac accessed 1 Feb 2025]

7. Open Data Dashboard of basic indicators Pan American Health Organization (PAHO). PAHO/EIH, 2021 [Available from: https://opendata.paho.org/es/indicadores-basicos/dashboard-of-basic-indicators accessed 22 Jan 2025]

8. Acting with a sense of urgency to prevent and end feminicides. Bulletin femicide violence in figures Latin America and the Caribbean. Gender Equality Observatory, ECLAC, 2024 [Available from: https://oig.cepal.org/es/documentos/boletin-violencia-feminicida-cifras-america-latina-caribe-ndeg3-actuar-sentido-urgencia accessed 1 Feb 2025]

9. Gregson K. Armed Violence and Programming for UNICEF in Latin America and the Caribbean: A Working Document. Panama: UNICEF, 2024.

10. Anderson MIP, Savassi LCM. 45 years of family and community medicine and 40 years of the Brazilian society of family and community medicine: Role, challenges and perspectives in the process of strengthening and qualification of primary care and the unified health system in Brazil. *Rev Bras Med Fam Comunidade* 2021;16(Suppl 1):7–17. https://doi.org/10.5712/rbmfc16(Suppl1)3244

11. Ponzo J. Family and community medicine in Uruguay from 1997 to 2019: How many kilometers will it take to reach that town? *Ciênc Saúde Collective* 2020;25(4):1205–14. https://doi.org/10.1590/1413-81232020254.29332019

CHAPTER 8

Exploring core values in family medicine in North America

David Ponka, Rodney Destine, Paula Henry, and Kim Yu

REGIONAL DESCRIPTION

The WONCA North American region (NAR) comprises two geographically large and populous high-income countries (HICs), the United States of America, population 345.4 million, and Canada, population 39.7 million, plus 11 sovereign island nations, 12 dependencies, and seven overseas territories in the Caribbean Sea (see Figure 8.1). The Spanish-speaking nations of Cuba and the Dominican Republic are considered part of the WONCA Iberoamericana-CIMF region.

The NAR Caribbean countries range from HIC to upper-middle-income (UMIC), with one (Haiti) low-middle-income country (LMIC). Many have very small populations of less than 1 million (Saint Kitts and Nevis at 47,000 to the Bahamas at 402,000), and three have larger numbers: Trinidad and Tobago, 1.5 million; Jamaica, 2.8 million; and Haiti, 11.8 million (see Table 8.1). The predominant religion is Christianity, and all countries have democratic governments, apart from Haiti, where an interim civilian government is in power.

North America and the Caribbean were colonized by European countries from the late 15th to the early 19th centuries, with the indigenous populations largely overcome. During this time European slave traders transported Africans to the region as an enslaved labour force. Many people in the

DOI: 10.1201/9781003542353-8

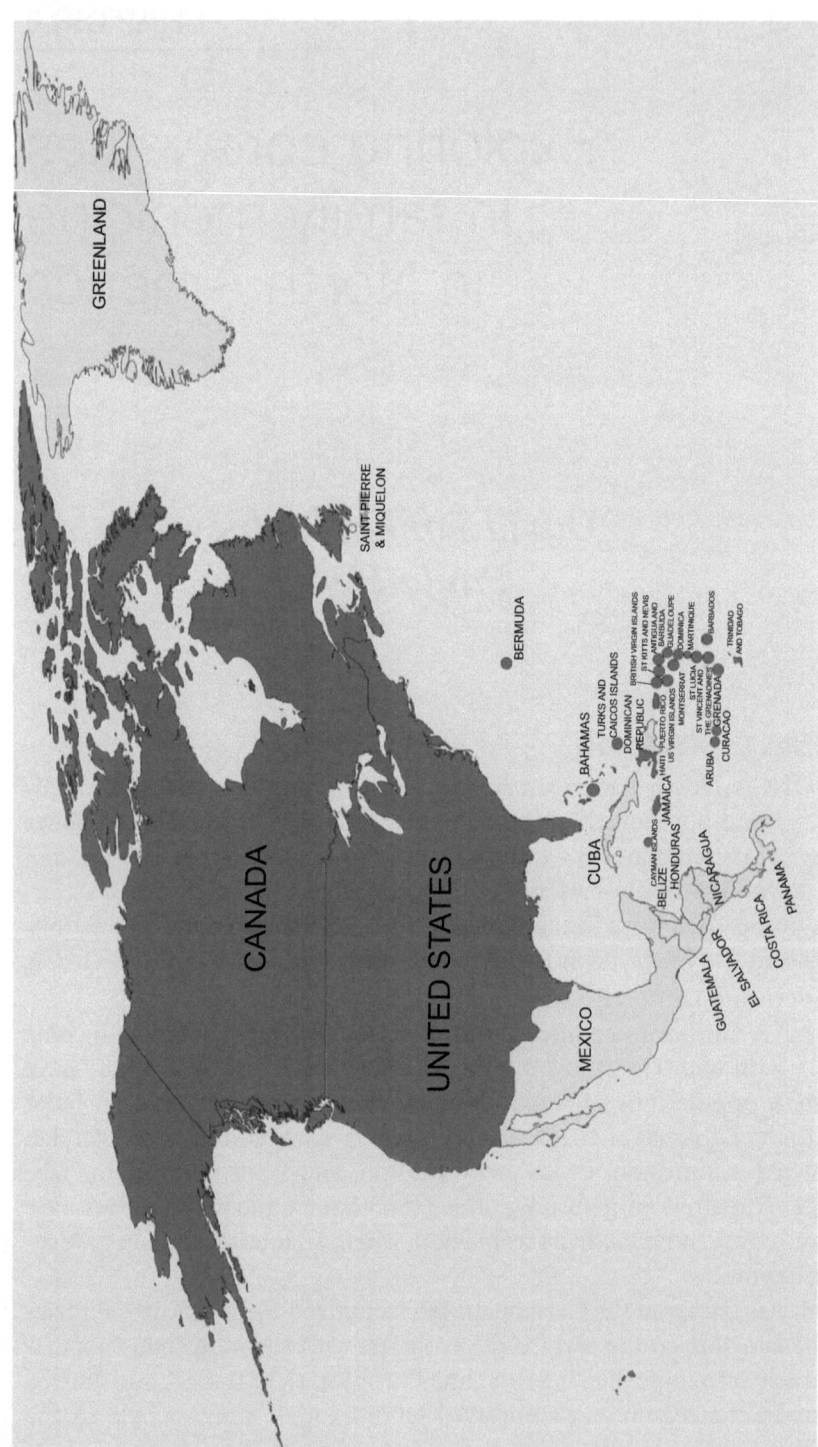

FIGURE 8.1 Map of the North American region.

Source: Map created with Mapchart.net

TABLE 8.1 Income Level and Population of Caribbean Countries

Caribbean Country	Income Level[1]	Population (2024)[2]
Antigua and Barbuda	HIC	93,772
Bahamas	HIC	402,168
Barbados	HIC	282,467
Cuba*	UMIC	10,700
Dominica	UMIC	66,205
Dominican Republic*	UMIC	11,427,557
Grenada	UMIC	117,207
Haiti	LMIC	11,772,557
Jamaica	UMIC	2,839,175
Saint Kitts and Nevis	HIC	46,843
Saint Lucia	UMIC	179,744
Saint Vincent and the Grenadines	UMIC	100,616
Trinidad and Tobago	HIC	1,507,782

* Spanish-speaking countries which are part of the WONCA Iberoamericana-CIMF region.

Caribbean and southern United States are of at least partial African descent. In the 19th century there followed an indentured labour system from India and China. More recent immigration has led to an increasing ethically and culturally diverse population in the region.

Factors contributing to values

In a very creative study during the COVID-19 pandemic, Grimalda and colleagues found that exposure to the virus increased charitable giving and sentiments of altruism amongst individuals.[3] The geographic level of altruistic action (giving to more local charities versus more globally minded ones) varied significantly, however, according to preestablished social identity: individuals in the United States were more likely to give to local or regional levels, whereas individuals in Italy were more likely to give at national or global levels. The authors posit that social identity lies closer to home in the United States than in Italy, perhaps because government agency is stronger at the individual state level in the United States, whereas agency and political decisions in Italy are made at the country or European level.

Political power in the Americas may be characterized by decentralisation and devolution, fostering local autonomy and diverse representation. While Canada is still a constitutional monarchy, health decisions are made at the provincial or territorial levels – it has been said that Canada has not 1 but 13 health systems (one for each of the 10 provinces and three territories). In the United States, healthcare delivery is complex and multifaceted, with a mix of private and public systems that can vary widely in terms of access, quality, and cost.

The Caribbean is still very much influenced by its colonial history. In no small part due to this, North America as a whole is amongst the most economically disparate regions of the world both within countries[4] and as a region, with Haiti being one of the most impoverished countries in the world.[5]

These normative influences and trends colour the health landscape and have influenced the establishment of family medicine (FM) on the continent. Canada established its first FM residency programme in 1966, followed by the United States in 1968. Both countries maintain a high number of family doctors and physicians per capita, and family doctors generally serve as gatekeepers in both healthcare systems, which are a combination of private and public elements, to help rationalise access to care. However, not all who live in Canada or the United States have access to their own family physician.

The Caribbean is diverse culturally, economically, and in how it utilises FM, where it is a newer concept. Barbados launched a three-year master programme in 1981.[6] Trinidad and Tobago has trained family physicians since at least the turn of the century, the Bahamas since 2002, St. Lucia since 2008, Jamaica since 2010, and Guyana since 2015. Haiti established a three-year residency programme in 2011, but it is currently not training residents due to internal conflict. The Caribbean region has a vocational family physician college established in 1987 (the Caribbean College of Family Physicians – CCFP) and which joined WONCA shortly thereafter.

The diversity within this region makes seeking foundational values of the discipline more important. This is especially true since we are still living in Tseng's fourth pandemic wave of moral and economic injury,[7] which is creating a tendency towards parochialism and polarization in society, including in the health workforce. Added to these challenges, looking forward, artificial intelligence (AI) has the potential to greatly disrupt health systems, making foundational, course-plotting values more important.

With these trends in mind, our work focuses less on the FM physician or practice-based values and more on the overarching health system–level values that borrow from, but also give back to, those of wider society.

PROCESSES

The selection of our team members was deliberate and based on maximum variation sampling to capture the widest range of perspectives possible, with the important inclusion of Haiti as an often-neglected Francophone voice in the region. Our process is an environmental scan of the diverse landscape of our region, done in two phases.

Phase 1

First, as a group of authors, we collected and collated the explicit values and principles of our respective organizations in an iterative, practice-informed approach. North America has a complex FM landscape. Of note, there are seven organizations representing family medicine in the United States: the American Academy of Family Physicians (AAFP), the Society of Teachers of Family Medicine (STFM), the American Board of Family Medicine (ABFM), the Association of Family Medicine Residency Directors (AFMRD), the American College of Osteopathic Family Physicians (ACOFP), the Association of Departments of Family Medicine (ADFM), and the North American Primary Care Research Group (NAPCRG). It is also important to note that Haiti is not officially a member of the CCFP, and the current conflict besieging that country presents a further challenge to capture data.

Note was made when a sub-organization or internal committee had declared values and values in action, such as The Besrour Centre for Global Family Medicine at the College of Family Physicians of Canada (CFPC). An effort was also made to understand and analyze both historical and current trends in the formation and adoption of FM at the context level, as well as current efforts at primary care practice reform. Values apparent through this analysis were recorded.

Phase 2

Second, we held a series of polls to inform the work. Virtual meetings were held in the Caribbean, and a workshop was held as part of a WONCA North America convening on 22 September 2024, in Phoenix, Arizona, held in conjunction with the AAFP Global Health Summit and FMX Annual Conference. A modified nominal group process[8] using live-polling technology was used to prioritize (1) values considered important to audience members, (2) potential applications of reasserting core values, and (3) possible barriers at the professional and societal level impeding these applications.

We also polled key leaders in Canada, the United States, and the Caribbean to inform our analysis of barriers and opportunities to emancipating FM's core values at this critical juncture for the discipline.

Finally, in the spirit of capacity building and participatory research, efforts were made to instil a sense of momentum and timeliness of opportunity after the polling of members, and we made our materials and processes available and free to use for other groups within the region.

FINDINGS

Phase 1

Document and website reviews of our respective organizations revealed that while mission and vision statements are well articulated, there was a paucity of explicit values amongst FM representative bodies in the region. Only the STFM, ADFM, and CFPC explicitly listed guiding values for their organizations, with the latter going further by listing examples of values in action or illustrations of how values should be applied.[9] Certain subgroups, for example, The Besrour Centre for Global Family Medicine, listed values (respect, excellence, equity, justice, reciprocity) which differed from those of their host organization, CFPC (respect, commitment to excellence, caring, learning, collaboration, responsiveness, integrity).[10]

Careful review of not only publicly available documents but also documents of subcommittees and working groups, informed by internal knowledge of the organizations, confirmed that values were often implicitly expressed within principles, projects, and strategic plans. For example, although several FM organizations such as the ABFM and the AAFP do not explicitly articulate values on their main webpages, their mission and strategic plans are replete with values, projects, and goals valuing professionalism, lifelong learning, and elevating FM standards, in addition to equity, advocacy, and collaboration.[11-13] The ADFM did also express values (excellence, integrity, inclusion, equity, respect, partnership) and ACOFP and NAPCRG also shared values within strategic plans online.[14,15]

Further analysis revealed a richness of implicitly embedded values. In the United States, FM organizations document key tenets of the specialty through the '2004 Task Force for the Future of Family Medicine',[16] defining core values as providing, 'continuing, comprehensive, compassionate, and personal care for their patients' and 'access to what is needed for people of any and all backgrounds and life circumstances' as well as being 'knowledgeable and willing to accept any type of problem and take responsibility either to provide the care or assure that care is provided by an appropriate source'. In addition, Phillips et al. note how the seven organizations developed a statement defining the family physician's role:

> Family physicians are personal doctors for people of all ages and health conditions. They are a reliable first contact for health concerns and directly address most health care needs. Through enduring partnerships, family physicians help patients prevent, understand, and manage illness, navigate the health system and set health goals. Family physicians and their staff adapt their care to the unique needs of their patients and communities. They use data to monitor and manage their patient population and use best science to prioritise services

most likely to benefit health. They are ideal leaders of health care systems and partners for public health.[17]

In addition, measures like the Person-Centered Primary Care Measure (PCPCM) developed by Etz, Stange, and ABFM and other measures of comprehensiveness of care and continuity are changing the way family physicians and primary care are evaluated and value the relationships that they provide to their patients.[18]

This practice-informed iterative group process is a taxonomy and hierarchy of core values in the region (Box 8.1). This includes some values (e.g. professional autonomy) that are not explicit in any documents but are nonetheless formative, considering the history of member interests and current attempts at practice reform.

Phase 2

Looking at the survey, there were 29 respondents attending remotely from the Caribbean and 42 in person in Phoenix. In both cases, these were exclusively

---

BOX 8.1 Taxonomy and hierarchy of core values in the region

EQUITY/SOCIAL ACCOUNTABILITY

Integrity

EMPATHY/COMPASSION

Relationship-based
Responsiveness
Respect
Diversity
Nurturing

PROFESSIONAL AUTONOMY

GENERALISM/ADAPTABILITY

Excellence
Lifelong learning

CONNECTION/COLLABORATION

Community-based
Openness

self-identified family physicians with a variety of backgrounds (practice focus, research, and academic leadership) from 12 countries.

Word clouds created from the live polling reveal a greater accordance of value prioritization in the Caribbean polls than in the poll held in the United States. In both polls, themes of equity, empathy, and connection/collaboration were considered most important.

Respondents felt the project was valuable and mostly cited applications for advocacy efforts, educational programmes, and identity formation in view of collaboration (Figures 8.2 and 8.3). Interestingly, policy change was not prominently cited as a potential use of the process. This may occur in part because barriers (Table 8.2) were largely considered to lie outside of the discipline, at the wider professional and societal levels.

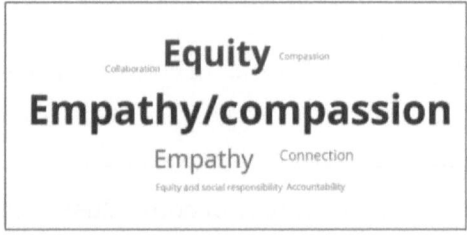

FIGURE 8.2 Word cloud from workshop held in the Caribbean.

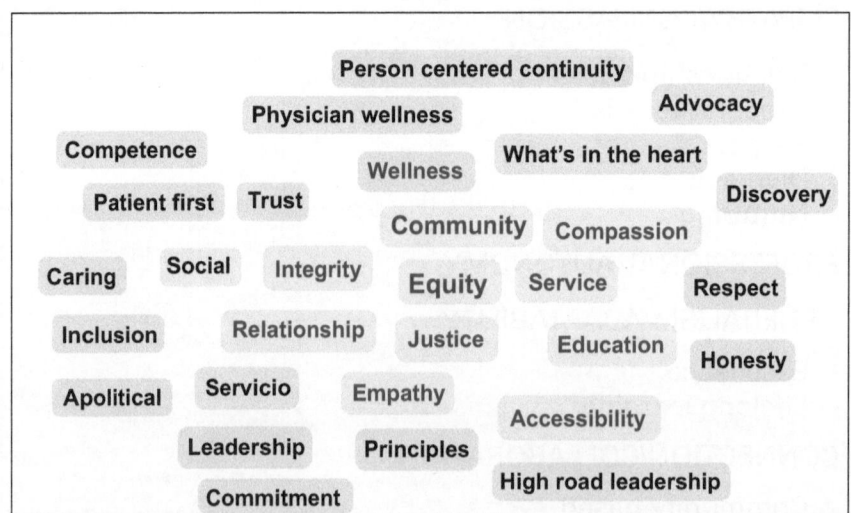

FIGURE 8.3 Word cloud from workshop held in the United States.

TABLE 8.2 Barriers to Adoption

Theme	Estimated Occurrences (N = 70)	%
1. Finance and pay inequities	14	20%
2. Burnout and moral injury	11	16%
3. Politics and external influences	11	16%
4. Healthcare system issues	9	13%
5. Racism and social disparities	7	10%
6. Insurance and regulations	5	7%
7. Devaluation and lack of recognition	5	7%
8. Lack of representation and advocacy	4	6%
9. Collaboration issues	2	3%
10. Hope and wellness	2	3%

IMPLICATIONS AND APPLICATIONS

FM lives in the liminal space between society and medicine. By definition a community-based first-contact service, family physicians feel a great influence from normative trends, and we can also bear a great impact on them. The current contentious climate of many sectors of society likely goes a long way in explaining the burnout and crisis in FM as well. That said, the fact that trainees are turning away from the discipline, leaving upwards of 20% of Canadian patients with no family doctor,[19] for example, is a trend that could have been predicted even before the pandemic.

Stange has argued that FM is at risk of ongoing compression if it continues to try and hold up a dysfunctional health system.[20] When asked about barriers to pursuing our foundational values, our respondents predominantly cited:

- Compensation and burnout as critical issues affecting healthcare professionals.
- Systemic and political barriers, including a broken healthcare system and political influences, as major obstacles.

- Racism and social inequities continue to hinder healthcare access and delivery, impacting the overall system.

We can also surmise some internal realities that present a challenge to fully emancipating our core values. These include:

- Division within the discipline, including between the realities of rural and urban physicians and from more members in general questioning the authority of organizing bodies.
- A tendency to silo educators and researchers within departments of FM, which risks making teaching less evidence-based and research less relevant to everyday practice.
- Less modeling of comprehensive practice, further exacerbating the trend of residents to choose more specialized, enhanced-skills types of practice.

Our respondents, however, saw reasons for optimism:

- Family physicians can contribute to advocacy, not only for their specialty but also for marginalised groups and policy reform.
- There is a strong interest in education and collaboration, which reflects a desire to both connect with others and guide the next generation.
- The identity and cohesion of family medicine are important, and several responses mentioned the need to celebrate core values and reinforce unity within the field.
- In the Caribbean there was an overarching sense of optimism and opportunity for FM. Respondents envisioned connectivity as the thread linking patients to physicians and physicians to each other and their fraternity. They envisioned the fraternity acting as a beacon, lending support, compassion, and empathy to its members.

Because of the diversity and disparity of the North American region, brief reports at the subregional level are useful. Canada is by default at the whim of the major societal and political trends of its more powerful neighbour. As a result, it has at times sought an international reputation as a fair arbitrator and a global influencer based on foundational and long-term values of tolerance, multiculturalism, and pluralism. Since the COVID-19 pandemic, however, a division has appeared within Canadian society itself – a polarization that has also affected the discipline of FM.

The CFPC has understandably, within a budgetary deficit and short-term framework, had to heavily prioritize pressing concerns of members: issues such as reducing administrative burdens, increasing support, and fair compensation. Investments such as curricular reform and global health have been recently de-emphasized: members have voted down a long-term project seeking to expand FM residency training to three years (from the current two – the shortest in the world), a reminder of the importance of professional autonomy and self-determination that have been at the heart of Canadian medical culture since its foundations. As another sign of local interests being prioritized, the College's global health centre has been defunded and has had to reorganize as an international network, risking isolating the Canadian health innovation landscape.

While Canada has one body representing FM (although with chapters at the provincial levels and helps oversee NAPCRG), the United States has seven, representing different aspects of the discipline. In both countries, these organizations work to promote comprehensive patient-centred care, advocate for the integration of social determinants of health, and emphasize the importance of continuous learning and professional development. They support the FM core values of comprehensiveness, continuity, and accessibility, advocating for a holistic approach to care that addresses both the physical and emotional needs of patients across the lifespan. By fostering a collaborative and multi-disciplinary environment, they also uphold the value of patient-centeredness, ensuring that FM practitioners are trained to build long-term relationships with their patients and communities.

Furthermore, these organizations emphasize the importance of social responsibility, working to reduce health disparities and improve healthcare access, especially in underserved areas. Their combined impact strengthens the FM field by promoting its commitment to advocacy, education, and quality care for all individuals, regardless of background or socioeconomic status. Results from our polling show that financial/pay inequities, as well as burnout and moral injury and political influences, are seen as barriers to adoption of core values. It is vital that organizations and the specialty of FM continue to work together to ensure that the core values of our specialty are firmly embedded. This requires a multifaceted approach to integrate these values into everyday practice and within health systems.

By creating an environment that values accessibility, continuity, and community engagement, family physicians and their organizations can ensure that these principles are not only taught but also consistently applied in everyday patient care, policy work, and healthcare delivery systems.

Colonial powers have shaped the region. The Caribbean takes its name from the Caribs, an ethnic group present in the Lesser Antilles and parts of the adjacent South America at the time of the Spanish conquest of the Americas in the 15th century. The modern Caribbean is ethnically diverse from colonization by the Spanish, English, Dutch, and French; the Atlantic slave trade from sub-Saharan Africa; indentured servitude from India and China; and modern immigration. In addition to the English, Spanish, French, and Dutch as primary languages, Creole and indigenous languages are also spoken.

Finances to support the public health system are based on the gross domestic product (GDP) of individual nation-states. For optimization of certain services, for example, primary percutaneous coronary intervention (PCI), economies of scale would mandate the development of regional centres, thereby increasing the ability of the region to benefit from emerging technologies. While the Caribbean has benefited from inputs from the Pan American Health Organization, the Inter-American Development Bank, and the Caribbean Public Health Agency, the success of quality primary care delivery has disproportionately rested on individual efforts of members.

The CCFP is the only member organization in the English-speaking Caribbean. Membership with the CCFP guarantees automatic membership into WONCA, albeit non-direct membership. Where nationalism trumps regional development, strong leadership in the CCFP could strengthen an enshrined FM value system.

Institutional training in the DM (Doctor of Medicine) and Diploma in Family Medicine in the currently five established campuses of the University of the West Indies has assisted in personal and academic advancement. Haiti, in contrast, is in an especially precarious position. Although FM training was established there in 2011, no training is currently occurring because of the violence the country is facing. As a result, FM is still not universally established or understood. It is a reminder that progress can never be taken for granted, nor does it always follow a predictable arc.

Preserving progress

FM is essential for providing comprehensive, continuous, and community-based care. In a resource-limited country like Haiti, where access to healthcare is often fragmented, FM ensures that individuals receive holistic care across the lifespan, from prevention to management of chronic diseases.

Haiti faces significant challenges in rural and underserved areas, where medical infrastructure is often lacking. FM training programmes are crucial because they prepare physicians to work in these settings, where they can provide critical care and build long-term relationships with communities. FM programmes contribute to the retention of healthcare providers in these areas, addressing the urban-rural disparity. By training doctors who are familiar with the local context, these programmes help ensure that health professionals are more likely to stay in the areas that need them most.

The progress made by the single FM training programme in Haiti is at risk due to funding cuts and sociopolitical instability. Its loss would mean the loss of a critical pillar of Haiti's healthcare system: it is crucial to reinforce advocacy as part of Haiti's broader effort to improve healthcare and develop local capacity. This can help garner much-needed support from local associations, governments, non-governmental organizations, and the international community.

FM residency programmes have the ethical responsibility to provide equitable healthcare access. In a country like Haiti, where social determinants of health (poverty, education, and access to clean water) pose significant challenges, ensuring access to quality primary care can have far-reaching effects on improving social and health outcomes.

Family physicians are often at the forefront in times of crisis, whether natural disasters, epidemics/pandemics, or political unrest. Ensuring a robust training system for family physicians equips Haiti with the capacity to be more resilient in the face of such challenges. To preserve Haiti's FM training programmes, it is crucial to emphasize not only their importance in addressing immediate healthcare needs but also their long-term impact on the country's health system and overall development. Preserving FM training programmes in Haiti is crucial for strengthening primary care access and ensuring long-term health system sustainability.

Highlighting the risks of losing this programme – such as reduced access to care, exacerbation of rural health disparities, and weakening of the healthcare workforce – demonstrates that preserving FM training is an investment in both the present and future of Haiti's healthcare landscape.

On a positive note, Haiti has a nascent national association representing family physicians – the Association Haitienne des Médecins de Famille (AHMEF).[21] Being primarily Francophone, Haiti does not enjoy WONCA membership on an otherwise mostly English- or Spanish-speaking continent. This Haitian organization would benefit from membership in WONCA to help preserve FM in this country in flux.

Unifying the landscape

Certain aspects of FM in North America illustrate a tendency towards devolution, if not fragmentation. This can have advantages in accounting for local realities but also consequences: missed opportunities for collaboration between disciplines or countries, for advocacy between rural and urban contexts, or for leverage between sectors such as primary care and public health that both have common goals.

Autonomy, collective organization/advocacy, and interdisciplinary collaboration perhaps are more related than we realise in that they lie on a spectrum. In the West, there is a tendency to think dualistically – in an and/or, zero-sum fashion. But while energies that strengthen professional autonomy can also strengthen the discipline, efforts to strengthen the discipline should ultimately be to strengthen the healthcare sector for the ultimate benefit of patients, and efforts across borders do not need to come at the expense of national priorities. In the post-pandemic context, we 'can and must do both'.[22]

A country can belong to two (or more) world regions, depending on classification. If form should follow function, perhaps institutional structures and governance can allow some flexibility with regard to this representation. For example, Cuba and Haiti could be allied to more than one WONCA region.

WONCA has two initiatives of particular interest to our respondents for the future: the youth movements (Polaris in North America) and the Rural Seeds initiative (also primarily students and young doctors, with an interest in rural issues). Both have the potential to unify landscapes and harness energy moving forward.

Riding the wave of momentum

Despite challenges, the region holds a lot of optimism for FM. The Caribbean in particular seems poised for a renewed valuation of 'low-tech, high-touch' care that can reignite momentum in the region. Currently, a great majority of patients report trusting their family physicians in the region, and this is largely based on personal connections that must not fall victim to overly managed or technology-dependent care.

This will require a conscious effort to stay united, not only across urban, rural and other divides but also across roles. FM teachers and researchers must work together to maintain the relevancy of the required evidence to implement change.

Above all, we need to maintain international connections. Parochial trends may be surprising occurring immediately after a global pandemic, which should remind us that everyone and everything are connected. However, it is usual in human history to look inwards and worry most about those closest to us when facing a crisis, until we realise that crises are becoming much more global in nature. At this time, what FM in North America needs more than anything is the hope that lies in our foundations and the promise that relationship-based care can carry us into the future.

CONCLUSION

St Exupéry famously wrote that what is most important is sometimes invisible to the eyes.[23] Likewise, certain core values are so influential and prevalent that they are either entrenched or assumed. Although FM is well established in our region, especially in Canada and the United States, it is part of a wider medical system that values specialization, technology, and intervention. Furthermore, the learned medical culture tends to be one where professional autonomy is not only valued but assumed.

Our region tends to encourage a political system where healthcare decision-making is made at the provincial or state levels, rather than national, let alone regional ones. The devolution of decision-making to the periphery and expectations of agency at the practice level set up a rich breeding ground for innovation but may make scaling up more challenging. Further full-scope qualitative research is needed to better understand why family physicians continue to believe in our founding values. It has also been interesting to reflect on why our regional core values are nuanced from European countries where welfare states, especially in northern Europe, are more prevalent. Two immutable realities may come into play. The first is historic: slavery and race relations throughout the region have challenged social harmony at times and hampered efforts at cohesion and common purpose.[24] Second, geographically, the Americas were colonized when land and space were abundant. This rewarded a frontier mentality marked by innovation and self-determination. Dissenters could always move farther away and, unlike in Europe where opinions, by geographic necessity, had to become more integrated, may have contributed to potential fragmentation, devolution, and autonomy becoming almost automatically valued.

The aspirational responses received in our surveys were not surprising considering the responder bias inherent in an environmental scan: respondents more likely to engage in such a process are more likely to be more idealistic as well. What was surprising was that only three out of nine official FM representative organizations in the region had explicitly recorded values, and only one described core values in action, that is, how core values could translate into everyday observable acts, although many did describe values in strategic plans and within the work done by family physicians.

Finally, we propose a meta-level reflection on this work itself, which can tell us about FM values, all authors in this book being family physicians. This has been an ambitious project and purposefully initially undefined to account for regional differences. This process has been successful based on personal connections and relationships, mirroring our values within a consultation room with a patient. But does it say that our principal survey occurred in a pre-workshop early on a Sunday morning was well attended? Can we imagine such a project gathering interest in other medical disciplines? It is hard to imagine.

This perhaps speaks to two enduring realities attached to the development of FM in our region and in others – the process of subspecialization that has led to a certain undercurrent of insecurity and vulnerability amongst generalists, and yet, engaged family physicians, at the core, seem to remain staunchly committed to preventing healthcare from becoming more transactional. Our respondents continue to emphasize core values including empathy, equity, and service.

Remaining regional variation can also reveal a truth about our discipline. Variation speaks not only to the need but also to the value of being able to adapt to local realities and changing times in order to keep serving our patients. Perhaps these reflections may spark discussion into the need for more explicit core values and a commitment to ensure that those are embedded in residency training into the future.

Core values are foundational but also meant to guide us in the long term. The regional youth movement of WONCA in North America is named 'Polaris' after the North Star and reminds us that we need guiding points to navigate the challenges ahead. Our discipline has never met a challenge as big as the one presented by AI. It has been said that while AI will not replace family doctors, family doctors who use AI will replace those who do not.[25] If done properly, the judicious use of AI will present an opportunity to focus on the overarching quality and core value of any good family physician – that of being human.

ACKNOWLEDGEMENTS

We acknowledge the contributions of Dr Clayton Dyck, Canada, for help with the iterative small group and survey portions of the project.

REFERENCES

1. The World Bank. World Bank Country and Lending Groups, 2025 [Available from: https://datahelpdesk.worldbank.org/knowledgebase/articles/906519-world-bank-country-and-lending-groups accessed Jan 2025]
2. Worldometer. World Population US, 2025 [Available from: https://www.worldometers.info/world-population/ accessed Jan 2025]
3. Grimalda G, Buchan NR, Ozturk OD, et al. Exposure to COVID-19 is associated with increased altruism, particularly at the local level. *Sci Rep* 2021;11(1):18950. https://doi.org/10.1038/s41598-021-97234-2
4. Board of Governors of the Federal Reserve System. Distribution of Household Wealth in the U.S. Since 1989 Washington DC [Available from: https://www.federalreserve.gov/releases/z1/dataviz/dfa/distribute/table/#quarter:129;series:Net%20worth;demographic:networth;population:all;units:shares]
5. World Bank Group. The World Bank in Haiti, 2024 [Available from: https://www.worldbank.org/en/country/haiti/overview accessed Jan 2025]
6. Global Family Medicine. North America/Non-Hispanic Caribbean: Wilfrid Laurier University, 2019 [Available from: https://globalfamilymedicine.org/region-overview-5]
7. Coates A, Fuad A-O, Hodgson A, et al. Health workforce strategies in response to major health events: A rapid scoping review with lessons learned for the response to the COVID-19 pandemic. *Hum Res Health* 2021;19(1):154. https://doi.org/10.1186/s12960-021-00698-6
8. O'Neill B, Aversa V, Rouleau K, et al. Identifying top 10 primary care research priorities from international stakeholders using a modified Delphi method. *PLoS One* 2018;13(10):e0206096. https://doi.org/10.1371/journal.pone.0206096 [published Online First: 2018/10/26].

9. The College of Family Physicians of Canada. Values in Action Mississauga, Canada, 2018 [Available from: https://www.cfpc.ca/CFPC/media/Resources/Communications/Values-in-Action.pdf accessed Dec 2024]

10. The College of Family Physicians of Canada. Besrour Centre for Global Family Medicine Community Mississauga, Canada: CFPC, 2024 [Available from: https://www.cfpc.ca/en/about-us/the-besrour-centre/about accessed Dec 2024]

11. American Board of Family Medicine. About ABFM Lexington, KY, USA: ABFM, 2024 [Available from: https://www.theabfm.org/about/ accessed Dec 2024]

12. American Board of Family Medicine. ABFM Strategic Plan Lexington, KY, USA: ABFM, 2024 [Available from: https://www.theabfm.org/about/strategic-plan/ accessed Dec 2024]

13. American Academy of Family Physicians. Who is the AAFP? Leawood, KS, USA: AAFP, 2024 [Available from: https://www.aafp.org/about.html accessed Dec 2024]

14. American College of Osteopathic Family Physicians. Strategic Plan Chicago, IL, US: ACOFP, 2024 [Available from: https://www.acofp.org/about/about-acofp/strategic-plan accessed Dec 2024]

15. North American Primary Care Research Group. NAPCRG Strategic Plan 2022–2025 Leawood, KS, US: NAPRG, 2022 [Available from: https://napcrg.org/media/2030/napcrg-strategic-plan_condensed_for-publication_1-2022.pdf accessed Dec 2024]

16. Task Force 1. Report of the task force on patient expectations, core values, reintegration, and the new model of family medicine. *Ann Fam Med* 2004;2(Suppl 1):134.

17. Phillips RL, Jr., Brundgardt S, Lesko SE, et al. The future role of the family physician in the United States: A rigorous exercise in definition. *Ann Fam Med* 2014;12(3):250–5. https://doi.org/10.1370/afm.1651 [published Online First: 2014/05/14].

18. Burch A. Implementing Comprehensive Care to Improve Outcomes Lexington, KY, USA: ABFM, 2024 [Available from: https://www.theabfm.org/implementing-comprehensive-care-to-improve-outcomes/ accessed Dec 2024]

19. Duong D, Vogel L. National survey highlights worsening primary care access. *Can Med Assoc J* 2023;195(16):E592–3. https://doi.org/10.1503/cmaj.1096049

20. Stange KC. Time for family medicine to stop enabling a dysfunctional health care system. *Ann Fam Med* 2023;21(3):202–4. https://doi.org/10.1370/afm.2981

21. Association Haitienne des Médecins de Famille. AHMEF Port-au-Prince, Haiti: AHMEF, 2024 [Available from: https://www.facebook.com/associationhaitiennedesmedecinsdefamille/ accessed Dec 2024]

22. Ponka D. A ridge in Southern Chad. *Can Fam Physician* 2024;70(11–12):746. https://doi.org/10.46747/cfp.701112746 [published Online First: 2024/12/06].

23. de Saint-Exupery A. The Little Prince. US: Reynal & Hitchcock 1943.

24. Alesina A, Glaeser EL. Why are welfare states in the US and Europe so different? What do we learn? *Horizons stratégiques* 2006;2(2):51–61. https://doi.org/10.3917/hori.002.0051

25. Robeznieks A. Why generative AI like ChatGPT cannot replace physicians: AMA, 2023 [Available from: https://www.ama-assn.org/practice-management/digital/why-generative-ai-chatgpt-cannot-replace-physicians accessed Dec 2024]

CHAPTER 9

Exploring core values in family medicine in South Asia

Sankha Randenikumara,
Raman Kumar,
Pramendra Prasad Gupta,
and Zainab Mohammad Anjarwala

REGIONAL DESCRIPTION

South Asia is the southern subregion of Asia, defined in geographical and ethnic-cultural terms. With a population of 2.04 billion, it contains a quarter (25%) of the world's population. The modern states of South Asia are Bangladesh, Bhutan, India, the Maldives, Nepal, Pakistan, and Sri Lanka (Figure 9.1).

There are eight member organizations (MOs) in WONCA, with some countries having two and others none (see Appendix). India, Pakistan, and Bangladesh have two MOs, Sri Lanka and Nepal have one, Bhutan does not have an MO but has an academic member in WONCA, and as yet there is no MO or academic membership in the Maldives.

Six of the seven countries are low-middle income (LMIC), with the Maldives upper-middle income (Table 9.1). India has the highest population at 1450 million, whereas the Maldives has the lowest at just over half a million. Despite the influence of urbanization, the majority of people in all seven countries live in rural areas, with the highest population density in the Maldives.

DOI: 10.1201/9781003542353-9

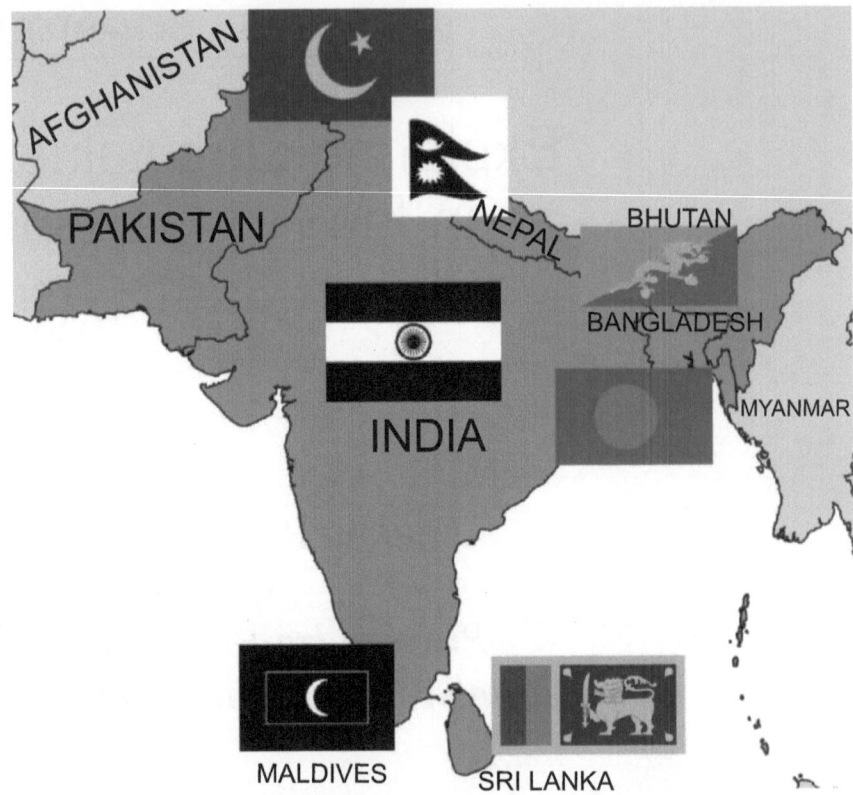

FIGURE 9.1 Map of the South Asia region with national flags.

Source: Map created with Mapchart.net

The religious composition of the South Asian region has been estimated to be 68% Hindu (concentrated in India and Nepal) and 31% Muslim (concentrated in Pakistan, Bangladesh, and the Maldives), with Buddhists (mainly in Sri Lanka and Bhutan), Jains, Zoroastrians, Sikhs, and Christians constituting most of the rest.[1]

No South Asian country has an established general practitioner (GP)/family physician (FP) referral system. Due to financial constraints, doctors with essential degrees (MBBS) have been legally permitted to practise in primary care as GPs, even though they do not have training in family medicine. However, in most of the countries, WONCA MOs and academia in family medicine have been involved in developing the discipline through undergraduate and postgraduate education. As a result, increasing numbers of trained FPs are practising in the community and academic institutions, although they have not yet received the due recognition. Many such trained FPs practise in the private sector and/or as part-time family doctors in many countries. Unfortunately,

TABLE 9.1 Demographic Data of the Countries in South Asia

Country	Income Group	Population	Population Density per km²	% Urbanization/ Rurality	Life Expectancy in Years	Unemployment % Total Labour Force
Bangladesh	LMIC	173,562,364	1333	42/58	74	5.1
Bhutan	LMIC	791,524	21	49.5/50.5	72	5.7
India	LMIC	1,450,935,791	488	36.6/63.4	68	4.2
Nepal	LMIC	29,651,054	207	23.8/76.2	71	4.7
Pakistan	LMIC	251,269,164	326	34.1/65.9	66	5.5
Sri Lanka	LMIC	23,103,565	368	17.9/82.1	77	6.4
Maldives	UMIC	527,799	1759	38.9/61.1	81	4.1

Sources:
The World Bank, https://datahelpdesk.worldbank.org/knowledgebase/articles/906519-world-bank-country-and-lending-groups
OECD/WHO. Health at a Glance: Asia/Pacific 2024, Paris, https://doi.org/10.1787/51fed7e9-en

there are no available data about people's access to trained FPs, as there is no differentiation between trained and untrained family doctors in the community.

BRIEF METHODS

We adopted three different methods to understand the interpretation and conceptualisation of core family medicine values in the South Asian region in the past and in the present.

Literature review of available resources in South Asia

A thorough literature review was conducted by searching all online material, such as WONCA MO websites and journal articles on core values. In addition, the core values group members reached out to MOs to find additional resources unavailable on the internet.

Survey on family doctors' views on core values

Using multiple methods for participant recruitment, an online questionnaire was circulated among the primary care doctors in the region. The questionnaire was piloted before being sent to online forums and MOs. The questions explored issues such as respondents' insights on traditional core values, challenges, new and emerging core values in a changing world, and cultural and socioeconomic relevance of core values. Incomplete responses were excluded, and data were analyzed using SPSS software using descriptive statistics.

Recording patient perspectives

A rapid literature review was conducted on patient perspectives on the values they expect from family doctors using the databases PubMed and Google Scholar. Articles published within the past ten years were searched using keywords 'family physicians', 'family doctors', 'general practitioners', 'patient perspectives', 'community perspectives', 'public opinion', 'patient expectations', and 'patient satisfaction'. Duplicates found in two databases were removed, and studies not related to South Asia were excluded. Full texts of the remainder were reviewed. Studies with a narrow scope (e.g., perspectives of home-based and palliative patients only) were excluded. There were nine papers in the final review.

FINDINGS

Insights from existing literature

Family medicine is a specialty that is vital in providing healthcare to rural and urban areas of South Asia, a region known for its distinct cultural background, economic challenges, and distinguishing healthcare needs. Although family medicine is a specialty recognized globally, its modification in South Asia echoes the unique goals and values of the region. From our review of studies conducted in the region and MO statements, several core values are shaped to suit this region's socioeconomic context: patient-centred care, accessibility, cultural sensitivity, continuity of care, and preventive health.

Patient-centred care actively involves patients in healthcare decision-making by identifying their desires, beliefs, and preferences. In South Asia, GPs/FPs frequently serve as primary healthcare providers, considering the social, cultural, and traditional factors that impact their health behaviours. This approach nurtures belief and adherence, particularly in areas where economic constraints and cultural taboos affect healthcare access.[2]

The social, economic, cultural, and geographical barriers make healthcare access extremely challenging for people in this region. Family medicine, however, promotes accessible care by developing community-based models that emphasize affordability and availability. These strategies often position FPs as primary healthcare providers in outreach programmes targeting underprivileged and rural communities. Hence, in areas with reduced access to specialists and advanced medical services, FPs may ensure that remote populations receive basic and advanced care.[3]

South Asia is one of the world's most linguistically, culturally, and religiously diverse regions. Cultural understanding is necessary for effective family medicine in this setting since patients' beliefs and customs significantly impact the healthcare decisions they make. In South Asia, FPs frequently modify their treatment methods to suit religious and cultural customs, like homeopathic or Ayurvedic treatments, which patients may prefer over conventional medical treatment. For example, the community-based *Vaidya* system, an ancient Indian tradition, referred to a local physician engaging with the population. The *Vaidya* tradition continues as the FP who engages with the community and provides cost-effective care with lifestyle changes, dietary advice, and traditional healing techniques.[4] This strengthens the doctor–patient relationship, as patients feel understood and valued in their cultural context.

A fundamental principle of family medicine is continuity of care, especially crucial for managing rising numbers of non-communicable diseases, including diabetes and cardiovascular disorders. Family medicine practices are central to providing thorough, continuous treatment, developing enduring connections which improve health outcomes.[5] FPs create a supportive atmosphere that improves patients' long-term health by offering individualised care, health education, and regular follow-ups. They frequently treat entire families spanning generations. They believe in a generalist approach, which involves treating the entire body irrespective of the organ or disease.[6]

In an area where infectious diseases such as malaria, dengue fever, and tuberculosis are common, preventive healthcare is crucial. To address these diseases, South Asian FPs strongly emphasize preventative measures such as immunization, health education, and cleanliness initiatives. Educating patients on lifestyle changes is another aspect of this focus to help counter the rise of non-communicable diseases in urban areas. In line with the comprehensive goal of family medicine, preventive health lowers healthcare expenditures. It promotes healthier societies, aligning with the prime objective of a holistic approach that every FP struggles to attain.[7]

South Asian family medicine has developed to incorporate ideals that align with the region's needs. In addition to improving healthcare results, these essential values tackle issues specific to South Asia, such as sociocultural diversity, economic inequality, and a lack of adequate healthcare infrastructure. The mission of family medicine in this region is driven by fundamental values such as patient-centred care, accessibility, cultural sensitivity, continuity, and preventative health, which guarantee that healthcare is practical, comprehensive, and respectful for various groups.

Most South Asian MOs have publications on values and principles, and each identifies different core values but with many common features (Table 9.2).

Analysis of survey

A total of 265 complete responses were analyzed. Maximum respondents were from India (76; 29%) followed by Sri Lanka (56; 21%), Nepal (51; 19%), Pakistan (46; 17%), Bangladesh (23; 9%), and Bhutan (13; 5%). One hundred and sixty-four (62%) were trained FPs, 34 (13%) were academics, 32 (12%) were trainees, 16 (6%) were untrained GPs, and 19 were (7%) non-GPs.

Traditional values
Respondents considered the following to be traditional core values: continuity of care (28%), patient-centred care (26%), holistic care (23%), comprehensive care (25%), coordinated care (16%), preventive care (15%), community-oriented care (12%), first-contact care (12%), compassionate care (11%), empathy (9%), and family-oriented care (9%). These core values were ranked highly by all the respondents who were trained FPs (Table 9.3). However, the understanding about traditional core values was lower among trainees, untrained GPs, and non-GPs. This demonstrates the importance of the family medicine postgraduate training for better clarity and understanding about the nature of the discipline.

New innovative values
New core values in family medicine in South Asia also emerged from the survey data. Respondents prioritized culturally sensitive patient-centred care, integrating respect for diverse traditions, beliefs, and family dynamics. They saw health equity as a cornerstone, ensuring accessible, affordable care

TABLE 9.2 Comparison of Core Values of Family Medicine/General Practice in South Asia

Core Value or Principle	Principles of Family Medicine by Riaz Qureshi, Pakistan (1998)[6]	Values in Family Medicine by College of General Practitioner Sri Lanka (2002)[8]	Principles of Family Medicine Academy of Family Physicians India (2010)[9]	General Practice (Family Medicine) in Nepal (2005)[10]	Domains of Family Medicine in Bhutan Curriculum (2016)[11]
Caring	Caring attitude	Gratitude	Care of patients in clinic, home, and hospital	Care of patients in clinic, home, and hospital	
Compassion	Compassionate care	Compassion	Understanding the context of illness	Compassionate care	
Comprehensiveness of care	Comprehensive care	Advocacy	Viewing the practice as a population at risk	Comprehensive care	Professional and ethical role domain
Coordination of care	Coordination of care	Decency	Commitment towards patients	Coordinated care	Organizational and legal dimension domain
Continuity of care	Continuity of care	Respect	Sharing with patients of same habitat	Continuity of care	
Preventive care	Common problems management	Loyalty	Practice preventive care Viewing the practice as a population at risk	Preventive care	

(Continued)

TABLE 9.2 (Continued)

Core Value or Principle	Principles of Family Medicine by Riaz Qureshi, Pakistan (1998)[6]	Values in Family Medicine by College of General Practitioner Sri Lanka (2002)[8]	Principles of Family Medicine Academy of Family Physicians India (2010)[9]	General Practice (Family Medicine) in Nepal (2005)[10]	Domains of Family Medicine in Bhutan Curriculum (2016)[11]
Doctor–patient relationship	Counselling and communication skills	Empathy	Recognition of the subjective aspects of medicine	Positive doctor–patient relationship	Communication and patient–doctor relationship
Competency	Clinical competence	Competence	Awareness of the need to manage resources	Applied professional knowledge and skills	Applied professional knowledge and skills
Cost-effectiveness	Cost-effectiveness			Cost effective care	
Community-based care	Community-based care and research		Use of community-wide network of supports	Community-based care	Community health and context of general practice

TABLE 9.3 Distribution of Respondents According to Their Opinion on Traditional Core Values

Core Value	Trained FPs		Academics		Trainees		Untrained GPs		Non-GPs		Total	
	N	%	N	%	N	%	N	%	N	%	N	%
Continuity of care	75	28	13	5	17	6	2	1	7	3	114	43
Patient-centred care	70	26	15	6	14	5	4	2	8	3	111	42
Holistic care	62	23	9	30	15	6	3	1	9	3	98	37
Comprehensive care	67	25	16	6	11	4	0	0	2	1	96	36
Coordinated care	44	17	12	5	13	5	4	2	3	1	76	29
Preventive, promotive . . .	39	15	9	3	7	3	1	0	5	2	61	23
Community-oriented care	31	12	6	2	5	2	2	1	2	1	46	17
First-contact care	32	12	7	3	5	2	1	0	0	0	45	17
Compassionate care	29	111	4	2	4	2	2	1	4	2	43	16
Empathy	25	10	5	2	4	2	1	0	4	2	39	15
Family-oriented care	24	9	6	2	3	1	3	1	1	0	37	14
Cost-effective	25	9	3	1	3	1	3	1.13	1	0	35	13
Ethics and professionalism	20	8	2	1	5	2	3	1	4	1.51	34	13

for underserved and marginalized populations. Community-oriented care should focus on preventive health, leveraging local resources and traditional practices to promote wellbeing.

The value of continuity of care can strengthen trust and long-term relationships within families and communities. Additionally, individual autonomy should balance with family involvement and collaborative decision-making, respecting the region's collective ethos. Embracing innovation, such as digital health tools (telemedicine, artificial intelligence [AI]), and addressing mental health and chronic disease stigmas are also vital for modernizing care while preserving cultural relevance.

Other values and principles to emerge included planetary healthcare (climate justice, environment sustainability), evidence-based decision-making, equity and inclusivity, advocacy and leadership, patient empowerment and shared decision-making, and cost-effectiveness.

Cultural aspects

In South Asia, cultural aspects deeply influence the core values of family medicine by emphasizing respect for traditions, family involvement, and community orientation. Patient-centred care requires understanding spiritual, social, and familial contexts, while long-term doctor–patient relationships align with the cultural emphasis on trust and personal connections. Addressing health disparities involves providing equitable, culturally competent care, especially to marginalized populations. Ethical practice balances individual autonomy with collective decision-making, reflecting family and community dynamics. Additionally, leveraging traditional practices for health promotion and addressing stigmas around mental health and chronic diseases are essential for effective, culturally sensitive healthcare delivery.

Responses received from the survey in priority order are:

- Personalized care, empathy, and respect – common core values could cater to the cultural differences, if used properly.
- Culturally sensitive (religious beliefs, sociocultural norms and values).
- Family involvement in care/family dynamics – family is the foundational and functional unit of South Asian civilization.
- Collectivism/collective decision-making.
- Respect for elders and wisdom.
- Gratitude.
- Community solidarity.
- Hospitality and compassion.
- Spiritual and holistic healing.
- Emotional expression and support.
- Trust and relationship building.

- Integrating traditional/alternative medical practices.
- Care for vulnerable populations, equity, justice.

Patient perspectives on core values

Recognizing patients' perspectives or expectations on the core values they seek in FPs is critical for improving healthcare delivery. The result of our rapid review found that patients' perspectives of values in FPs among South Asians focuses on compassion, social beliefs, communication, trust, and respect. The doctor–patient relationship is very important, as that greatly influences healthcare interactions. We report the findings from the nine papers in our review.

Compassion is essential for quality healthcare and is fundamental to bridging cultural and ethnic differences between patients and their healthcare providers. Singh et al. found that South Asian patients considered compassion a key component of quality healthcare. The researchers recommended overcoming language and cultural barriers to providing compassionate care to patients.[12]

Patient satisfaction is one of the cardinal facets of healthcare initiatives by any nation. Providing high-quality services is indispensable for the success of any service provider. Patients' experiential values, both extrinsic and intrinsic factors, eventually impact how patients assess the quality of healthcare they receive. A study in India by Dhal et al. reported that various intrinsic qualities such as belief, trust, safety, convenience, and accessibility can be adopted by an FP to increase patient-centred care.[13] Another study from India emphasized the role of empathetic behaviour in effective healthcare delivery, as it positively influences the physician–patient relationship, leading to better outcomes.[14]

A study in Pakistan by Irshad et al. reported that most patients value doctors who treat them with care, respect, and dignity. The physician should be able to explain the condition and answer questions in ways that patients can understand.[15] In Sri Lanka, quality of care is similar in both public and private sectors, with patients perceiving better physicians to be those who are competent, as well as having good communication and interpersonal skills.[16]

Bangladesh is a country dealing with cultural differences, illiteracy, and diverse religious and social norms, and hence, it has multifaceted scenarios of patient–physician relationships. In a study on patients' views on physicians' communication skills in telemedicine, it was found that patients valued being treated with respect, being allowed to talk without interruption, and having physicians spend a sufficient amount of time with them.[17] Another study reports that physicians who respect the autonomy of the patients and provide ethical care as their moral basis were considered to have an ideal patient–physician relationship.[18]

In Nepal, where most of the population resides in rural areas, primary care physicians are important in providing access to basic healthcare needs. A study by Stone found that recognition of community participation in Nepal's traditional medical system and respect for patients' own ideas and values would help improve patients' engagement with healthcare.[19] Another study reported that Nepalese patients prefer being treated by respectful, friendly, knowledgeable physicians who give sufficient consultation time and practise preventive care. They preferred the doctor to take charge and did not want a shared decision-making approach.[20]

In summary, South Asian patients broadly value FPs who practice with compassion, empathy, competence, accessibility, and cultural sensitivity. Although various challenges exist, such as resource limitations and systemic inefficiencies, FPs who prioritize trust-building, clear communication, and ethical practices often stand out optimistically in patient perspectives.

IMPLICATIONS AND APPLICATIONS

A statement on core values in family medicine in 2025 could be highly beneficial for clinicians in South Asia, as it would provide a clear framework for delivering patient-centred care in diverse and resource-constrained settings. These core values will reinforce the importance of long-term doctor–patient relationships, which align with traditional trust-based practices in South Asia. It will emphasize respect, empathy, and confidentiality, helping clinicians navigate complex cultural and ethical challenges. Treating patients as individuals within their family and community contexts is a key aspect of South Asian healthcare. Furthermore, it will encourage judicious use of limited resources, emphasizing prevention, early diagnosis, and cost-effective interventions. There is an unmet need to reduce disparities and improve access to care for marginalized populations, addressing a pressing regional challenge. Finally, core values will serve as a foundation for continuous learning and reflective practice for clinicians. Such a statement could unify clinicians around shared goals, improve patient outcomes, and elevate the standards of primary care in the region.

Implementing core values in family medicine in South Asia faces barriers at multiple levels due to systemic, cultural, and individual challenges. At the national level there are policy gaps. There is a lack of robust policies prioritizing primary healthcare and family medicine as a specialty. There is insufficient government investment in healthcare infrastructure and training for FPs. There is an existing rural–urban divide as an outcome of disproportionate resource allocation, leaving rural areas underserved. There is poor integration of primary, secondary, and tertiary care, limiting continuity of care. Furthermore, there is weak enforcement of ethical and professional standards in medical practice. At the regional level there is significant variation in resources, workforce distribution, and healthcare accessibility across regions. There are diverse cultural norms and beliefs that may conflict with standardized medical practices or core values.

Scarcity of family medicine training programmes in countries hinders capacity-building. This gap has been used by several profit-oriented programmes, which do not focus on providing community need–based, country-specific training in some countries. Frequent disruptions due to conflict or governance issues also affect healthcare delivery. At the individual level over-burdened clinicians face time constraints, limiting their ability to focus on holistic and preventive care. There is a lack of awareness or formal education in family medicine among GPs, and established practitioners may be reluctant to adopt new frameworks or practices. High workload, limited support, and challenging conditions undermine clinicians' ability to adhere to core values. Financial incentives often favour specialty or procedural care over comprehensive, patient-centred care. Core values in family medicine are often not implemented when planning undergraduate and postgraduate curricula and research projects.

Addressing these barriers requires systemic reforms, robust advocacy, investment in training and infrastructure, and cultural shifts to integrate family medicine values into practice effectively.

CONCLUSION

Family medicine and FPs play a crucial role in the healthcare systems of South Asia, characterized by a unique set of core values that guide their practice. These values are essential as they navigate the complexities and diverse healthcare needs of this region, home to a significant portion of the world's population. The core values and principles of family medicine in South Asia include comprehensive care, continuity of care, patient-centredness, community orientation, and cultural sensitivity. In family medicine, comprehensive care addresses the broad spectrum of patients' health issues.

FPs are often the first point of contact in the healthcare system, providing a wide range of services from preventive care to treating acute and chronic conditions. This comprehensive approach is crucial in a region where healthcare resources can be limited and access to specialists may be constrained. FPs manage various health problems, ensuring patients receive holistic healthcare that considers physical, mental, and social factors. Continuity of care is another cornerstone principle, emphasizing the ongoing relationship between FPs and their patients. This is significant in South Asia, where strong family and community ties are prevalent. FPs often serve multiple generations within the same family, fostering trust and understanding over many years. This long-term relationship enhances the quality of care as physicians gain in-depth knowledge of patients' health histories, vital for effective diagnosis and treatment. Continuity of care also supports better management of chronic diseases prevalent in the region due to changing lifestyles and increasing longevity.

Patient-centred care is integral to family medicine in South Asia, focusing on patients' individual needs and preferences. Recognizing that every patient is unique, FPs prioritize listening to patients, respecting their values, and involving them in decision-making. In the culturally diverse societies of South Asia, this approach ensures that care is tailored to align with cultural, spiritual, and personal beliefs. This value helps build trust and encourages patients to engage actively in their health management, which improves adherence to treatment plans and overall health outcomes.

FPs have the potential to contribute significantly to improving public health in South Asia, where the burden of communicable and non-communicable diseases is high, by focusing on community-level health promotion and disease prevention. Cultural sensitivity is paramount. FPs operate in environments where cultural practices and beliefs can significantly influence health behaviours and healthcare perceptions. By understanding and respecting these cultural nuances, FPs can provide effective, respectful, and acceptable care to patients. This sensitivity extends to communication styles, traditional health practices, and the involvement of family members in healthcare decisions, ensuring that medical interventions are culturally congruent and ethically sound.

These values and principles guide FPs in providing quality care to individual patients and empower them to act as vital contributors to the overall health and wellbeing of the communities they serve. As South Asia continues to develop, family medicine will remain indispensable in addressing the region's diverse healthcare needs.

ACKNOWLEDGEMENTS

Our thanks to the members of the South Asian core values team: Hina Jawaid (Pakistan), Chhabhi Lal Adhikari (Bhutan), Kinley Bhuti (Bhutan), Kabir Khan (Bangladesh), Ramakrishna Prasad (India), Aishana Joshi (Nepal), Shyamalee Samaranayake (Sri Lanka), and Paramita Karim (Bangladesh) for their helpful contributions.

REFERENCES

1. Pew Research Center. Table: Religious Composition by Country, in Numbers: The Pew Charitable Trusts, 2010 [Available from: http://www.pewforum.org/2012/12/18/table-religious-composition-by-country-in-numbers/ accessed Jan 2025]
2. Mudiyanse RM. Need to teach family medicine concepts even before establishing such practice in a country. *Asia Pac Fam Med* 2014;13(1):1. https://doi.org/10.1186/1447-056x-13-1 [published Online First: 2014/01/09].

3. Anam A, Ullah M. Effectiveness of community clinics in primary healthcare in Bangladesh: An empirical study. *Dyn Public Adm* 2021;38(1):28–42.

4. Kumar R. The 'Vaidya' – the ancient Indian family physician: The origin of family medicine specialty in India – a call for action by the National Medical Commission (NMC). *J Fam Med Prim Care* 2024;13(2):397–400. https://doi.org/10.4103/jfmpc.jfmpc_266_24 [published Online First: 2024/04/12]

5. Jawaid H, Prasad R. Promoting South Asian primary care research and projecting family medicine practitioner-scholars: A matter of critical importance. *J Fam Med Prim Care* 2023;12(10):2197–200. https://doi.org/10.4103/jfmpc.jfmpc_1530_23 [published Online First: 2023/12/11]

6. Hashim MJ. Principles of family medicine and general practice – defining the five core values of the specialty. *J Prim Health Care* 2016;8(4):283–7.

7. Porter J, Boyd C, Skandari MR, et al. Revisiting the time needed to provide adult primary care. *J Gen Intern Med* 2023;38(1):147–55. https://doi.org/10.1007/s11606-022-07707-x [published Online First: 2022/07/02]

8. College of General Practitioners of Sri Lanka. Advising Ourselves about Values in Family Medicine: CGPSL, 2002.

9. Kumar R. Vision, mission, goals, and objectives of the academy of family physicians of India. *J Fam Med Prim Care* 2024;13(6):2181–2. https://doi.org/10.4103/jfmpc.jfmpc_936_24

10. Lewis M, Smith S, Paudel R, et al. General practice (family medicine): Meeting the health care needs of Nepal and enriching the medical education of undergraduates. *Kathmandu Univ Med J* 2005;3(2):194–8.

11. Adhikari CL. Curriculum for masters in general practice – Bhutan. *J Fam Med Prim Care* 2021;10(6):2061–119. https://doi.org/10.4103/jfmpc.jfmpc_1727_20

12. Singh P, King-Shier K, Sinclair S. South Asian patients' perceptions and experiences of compassion in healthcare. *Ethn Health* 2020;25(4):606–24. https://doi.org/10.1080/13557858.2020.1722068

13. Dhal A, Sharma A. Exploring patient's experiential values and its impact on service quality assessment by Indian consumers in public health institution: A qualitative study. *J Public Aff* 2022;22(S1):e2800. https://doi.org/10.1002/pa.2800

14. Borkar SM. Empathy in physician–patient relationship: The construct and its applicability to India's health care. *Soc Change* 2014;44:423–38.

15. Irshad HA, Mahar MU, Jahangir A, et al. An assessment of public experiences and expectations with physicians: A cross sectional study from Karachi, Pakistan. *BMC Health Serv Res* 2024;24(1):108. https://doi.org/10.1186/s12913-023-10519-2

16. Rannan-Eliya RP, Wijemanne N, Liyanage IK, et al. The quality of outpatient primary care in public and private sectors in Sri Lanka – how well do patient perceptions match reality and what are the implications? *Health Policy Plan* 2015;30(Suppl 1):i59–i74. https://doi.org/10.1093/heapol/czu115

17. Islam MA, Hasan T, Mostari S, et al. Patients' views on physicians' communication skills in telemedicine: Validation of communication assessment tool among Bangladeshi sample. *J Commun Healthc*: 1–10. https://doi.org/10.1080/17538068.2024.2438474

18. Ahmed T. The case of doctor-patient relationship in Bangladesh: An application of relational model of autonomy. *BJBio* 2021;12(1):14–24. https://doi.org/10.3329/bioethics.v12i1.51900

19. Stone L. Primary health care for whom? Village perspectives from Nepal. *Soc Sci Med* 1986;22(3):293–302. https://doi.org/10.1016/0277-9536(86)90125-5

20. Moore M. What does patient-centred communication mean in Nepal? *Med Educ* 2008;42(1):18–26. https://doi.org/10.1111/j.1365-2923.2007.02900.x

CHAPTER 10

Review of the core values in our regions

Anna Stavdal, Johann Agust Sigurdsson, and Felicity Goodyear-Smith

REVIEW OF THE REGIONS

WONCA's mission is 'to improve the quality of life of the peoples of the world through defining and promoting its values, including respect for universal human rights and including gender equity, and by fostering high standards of care in general practice/family medicine'.[1] The aim of this Global Core Values project is to conduct an ongoing brainstorming and reflective process on core values and principles and the definition of the specialty of family medicine.

In the preceding chapters, our regional leaders and their teams have explored core values in family medicine, each in their own way, seeking the views of their family medicine colleges and other institutions and of family medicine doctors working on the ground in a diverse range of countries in their respective regions. While different regions have included research elements such as surveys and interviews to inform their work, overall this is not a research project per se; rather, we consider it to be a global enquiry. We have reviewed and identified some of the key points from their work.

Africa

Sub-Saharan Africa consists of 48 countries, of which 23 are low income and only one is high income. There are 3000 registered family physicians in 12 countries serving a total population of 916 million. Realistically, most people cannot have their own family doctor, who mostly work in district hospitals

DOI: 10.1201/9781003542353-10

providing general medical care. First-contact care is provided by community-based nurses and other primary care workers, who refer patients to family physicians as needed. In their explorations in this project, our African colleagues found the usual important family medicine core principles are continuity of care (to counter the focus on vertical programmes in secondary and tertiary care), coordination, and comprehensiveness. They identified family medicine core values as person-centredness, using the patient's agenda to drive the consultation, a family and community rather than an individual orientation, awareness and respect for cultural identity, advocacy to strengthen health systems, and lastly compassion, which drives all the other values in an effort to provide quality care for all patients.

Asia Pacific

The Asia Pacific region too contains a huge range of countries, from China covering 9.6 million square kilometres and a population of over 1.4 billion, to tiny island states in the Pacific Ocean with populations in the 100,000s and areas of less than 1000 square kilometres, such as the Kingdom of Tonga. They range from high-income countries (HICs) such as Australia and New Zealand to low-middle-income countries such as Myanmar and include Muslim, Christian, Buddhist, and secular states. The Asia Pacific team managed to gather data from a diverse sample of countries and integrated their overarching themes from both member organizations and their family doctor workshop to provide a unifying vision for family medicine in Asia Pacific. Similarly to Africa, they identified the most important core values to be patient-centred holistic care; building strong, trusting relationships through empathy and compassion; the integration of family and community healthcare delivery; and emphasis on prevention, early intervention, and long-term wellness. They see this as just the beginning of a process of exploration and iterative feedback.

East Mediterranean

The East Mediterranean Region (EMR) faces huge challenges. Many countries are wracked by war, millions of people are displaced resulting in huge refugee populations, and there are humanitarian challenges to address profound poverty and disruption of essential services such as healthcare provision and education. However, EMR also includes the HIC oil-rich Arab states of the Persian Gulf. Despite countries' differing cultural, social, and economic contexts and the diverse healthcare challenges, the region has 14 core values and principles as aspirational, with the goal of fostering a cohesive and resilient primary care system. Strengthening the family medicine discipline will help address the unique and evolving health needs of their diverse populations.

Europe

The area covered by WONCA Europe is vast, extending from the Arctic Ocean to the Mediterranean Sea, the North Atlantic Ocean to the west, and the Pacific Ocean to the east. It includes places usually considered Asian (Eastern Russia, Central Asian countries), as well as those traditionally considered part of the Western world (along with North America and Australasia), with a myriad of languages and cultures.

As outlined in Chapter 2, WONCA Europe had already endorsed core values for their region in 2022,[2] and their processes for this project focused on determining whether family physicians recognized these established core values in their countries and whether they implemented them in their daily practice. While they view their published core values and principles as an inspiration for other regions of the world, they also concede that core values may differ elsewhere and a review of these might lead to an update of their own. They are the first WONCA region to include planetary health on their agenda.[2]

Latin America

This region focuses on the Spanish- and Portuguese-speaking countries of Central and South America and the Caribbean. The region is characterized by a significant proportion of the population living in poverty, especially children; high rates of homicide; and armed conflicts, with governmental instability in many of the countries. However, there is also natural and cultural diversity and a large number of indigenous peoples with different cultures and languages. The WONCA Ibero-Americana regional group developed from the pre-existing Ibero-American Confederation of Family Medicine (CIMF), which includes Spain and Portugal (covered in the European chapter in this book). The Latin American authors have summarized the eight family medicine summits that have taken place in the region over two decades and extracted key values and principles from their published charters. They also plan to interview key stakeholders in the future.

North America

In contrast, the North American region is dominated by the two large, populous HICs of the United States and Canada, plus 11 small island countries in the Caribbean, ranging from affluent ones such as the Bahamas to the poverty-stricken and politically unstable Haiti. This regional group identified the fact that their landscape is characterized by decentralisation and devolution, fostering local autonomy to account for diversity. While empathy and compassion were seen as core values, the emphasis was often on issues of equity, social accountability, and professional autonomy.

South Asia

A quarter of the world's population resides in the combined seven countries of South Asia. The South Asian team explored core values and principles of family medicine from the three perspectives of the member organizations, family doctors themselves, and their patients. What emerges clearly in this chapter is the importance of family and how the Western concept of individual autonomy needs to be tempered by family involvement in a patient's care and decision-making. Similar to the African and Asia Pacific regions, the authors emphasize the importance of respecting cultural values and beliefs and the collective family-orientated ethos of the region.

WHAT DOES THIS REVIEW TELL US?

People from different countries, ethnicities, cultures, and beliefs hold different values and principles. Values reflect distinct cultural orientations. For example, Western values tend to be individualistic, with a focus on personal autonomy, independence and uniqueness, self-realisation, individual rights, and justice, and a competitive spirit is encouraged.

The core cultural values of Polynesian people from Pacific Island nations contrast sharply with those of the 'West'. They are about family and kinship; collectivism and communitarianism involving teamwork, collaboration, and cooperation; spirituality; reciprocity; and respect and humility.[3] There is interdependence, with a focus on mutual support and cooperation, maintaining good relationships and avoiding conflict, and a collective responsibility, with success measured by the wellbeing of the community rather than individual achievements. Cultural heritage and customs are preserved and respected. In Māori culture, societal lore (*tikanga*) provides behavioural guidelines for living and interacting with others.[4] Traditional values protect the wellbeing of the family (*whānau*) and survival of the collective. Core values are caring for those around us in the way we relate to each other (*manaakitanga*), recognizing the importance of kinship and lasting relationships (*whanaungatanga*) and the connection between people and the natural world (*kaitiakitanga*). We must be guardians of the natural environment to look after resources and ensure their survival for future generations.

In Africa, these Polynesian values are similarly reflected in their emphasis on family and community and cultural awareness. Asia Pacific and South Asia also recognize the importance of building strong, trusting relationships through empathy and compassion and integrating family and community services. North America, on the other hand, focuses on Western values of equity, social accountability, and autonomy, and the European core values and principles have largely been developed through the consensus of Western countries.

In a study comparing how family medicine is practised in various countries, Meads et al. recognized the adaptability of primary care and its manifestation in different sociopolitical contexts and identified different forms of practice organization in response to resources and needs of the population.[5] Western individualistic cultures value personal freedom, self-sufficiency, and independence, and competition and striving to achieve are important. In contrast, Eastern cultures may be more collectivist, meaning people are seen as fundamentally connected to and interdependent on other. Life is more family focused, and collective decision-making and reciprocity are valued. Our South Asian colleagues point out that the patient-centred model may not sit well with people whose culture involves the family involved in decision-making for a patient and who defer to the authority of their healer to make the best decision on their behalf. Clearly there are values common to all – that family doctors treat all with empathy and compassion, but the family medicine core values and principles of countries and regions may need to be adapted to match the communities they serve.

REFERENCES

1. WONCA. WONCA in Brief Bangkok, 2013 [Available from: http://www. globalfamilydoctor.com/AboutWonca/brief.aspx accessed Jul 2015]
2. WONCA Europe. The European Definition of General Practice/Family Medicine, 2002:35. (Edition 2023)
3. Ofanoa M, Paynter J, Buetow S. 'O'ofaki: A health promotion and community development concept to bring Pasifika people together. *Health Promot Internation* 2021;36(1):3–7. https://doi.org/10.1093/heapro/daaa025
4. Ofanoa M, Pau'uvale A, Goodyear-Smith F. Chapter 1: Who are the pacific people? In: Ofanoa M, Goodyear-Smith F, eds. Pacific Health Community Engagement: How to Do It with Diverse Pacific Communities in the Pacific and in Aotearoa New Zealand 2025.
5. Meads G, Wild A, Griffiths F, et al. The management of new primary care organizations: An international perspective. *Health Serv Manag Res* 2006;19(3):166–73. https://doi. org/10.1258/095148406777888125

CHAPTER 11

Core values to inspire global change

Anna Stavdal, Johann Agust Sigurdsson, and Felicity Goodyear-Smith

THE NATURE OF VALUES

As we determined in our first chapter, our personal values are deeply held beliefs about what is important, good, right, or wrong. They shape our attitudes and drive our actions and judgments.

At a different level, the guidelines and standards we create to ensure consistency, quality, and safety in how we practise – our processes and service – also guide our behaviour and decision-making. On the surface these appear objective, but our values are embedded within them.[1] They are often developed based on shared values to ensure that the outcomes align with what is considered important and beneficial, but as such may serve the interests of some groups at the expense of others. It is important therefore to continually reconsider what are the core values and principles which imbue our guiding documents. Fulford writes that the counterpart of evidence-based medicine is values-based medicine.[2] Where there may be complex and conflicting values, the processes of values-based practice enable balanced decision-making within a framework of shared values.[3] Whereas codes of practice prescribe good outcomes, value-based medicine focuses on the importance of good processes.[2]

Note that values-based practice is about values we hold important and to which we attribute worth, which serve as guides to action. This is to be differentiated from value-based healthcare, which is about getting the best value for money for the available resources in a way that is equitable, sustainable, and transparent to achieve better outcomes and experiences for every person.[4]

DOI: 10.1201/9781003542353-11

Professional values can be considered at three levels. Values-based practice operates at the micro level of the consultation and provision of healthcare for individuals. It focuses on the interactions of practitioners and patients and their families.

At the meso level there is an extended multi-disciplinary primary care team who has a diverse range of skills, and their disciplines may operate under a range of different values. The diverse values in play in a given situation need to be identified and a balanced decision made about what is to be done. Conflicting values need to be resolved either by consensus or by dissensus, where differences in values are resolved one way or another depending on context in an environment of mutual respect.[5]

While we need to be cognisant of the individual values of the family physician and of the primary care team that drives their behaviour, this global project is operating at the macro level of national organizations – their vision and mission – exploring the nature of the discipline of family medicine and the core values and principles of the profession in countries, regions, and around the world.

THE NATURE OF GENERALISM

Primary care physicians are often considered to provide poorer-quality care for specific diseases when compared to specialists. However, overall, primary care is associated with higher-value healthcare at the level of the whole person and better health, greater equity, lower costs, and better quality of care at the level of populations.[6] This is described as the paradox of primary and generalist care.

Generalists operate under three simple rules: (1) they recognize and make sense of problems and opportunities; (2) they prioritize their attention and action towards promoting health, healing, and personal connection; and (3) they personalize care based on the particulars of the person in their family and community context. Their interactions are largely relational. In contrast, specialists (1) identify and classify disease or management, (2) interpret their findings through specialized knowledge, and (3) manage a plan for disease care.[7] In general they provide transactional care. Naturally, generalists will also operate under these specialist rules, providing evidence-based care of single diseases in an individual patient for both acute and chronic illness.[8]

Stange writes that the generalist way is being open, humble, and connected, of knowing both the whole person and particulars of their health and wellbeing. Generalists scan, prioritize, and then focus on particulars while keeping the whole person in view. Their thinking and their actions involve contextualizing, connecting, and integrating what they know and learn.[6] As generalists, they attend to multiple problems and undifferentiated illness, deal with prevention and mental health issues, looking after individuals but also families, the community, and the population under their care.[8] Family medicine is about continuity, investing in relationships, having generalist knowledge and personal ways of knowing. There may be competing opportunities in patients with many issues and problems that might be addressed at some time, and the 'guideline' approach may not be the best course of action in the overall context of their physical, mental, social, and spiritual health at that time.

CONTINUITY AND COMPREHENSIVENESS OF CARE

Barbara Starfield emphasized the importance of continuity and comprehensiveness of care as two of the key attributes of primary care. Better health outcomes occur when a family doctor provides holistic first-contact care for the full range of a patient's health needs and has a consistent and ongoing relationship with a patient, building trust and better communication.[9]

However, this is often not an achievable goal. In regions such as Africa, the luxury of one's 'own' family doctor is unattainable, at least for most people in the population, and family doctors act as consultants in district hospitals, with nurses and other primary care workers out in the field.

For many living in countries in Europe, North America, and Australasia, having your own general practitioner from cradle to grave, your first-contact healthcare provider for all your needs, is no longer a reality. Especially in urban areas, primary care is fragmented. There is now a multiplicity of primary care providers. General practitioner services may be replaced by midwives who provide antenatal care and deliver the babies, family planning clinics provide contraception, sexual health centres provide tests and treat sexually transmitted infections, and urgent care clinics cater for people with injuries and acute medical issues. Instead of out-of-hours home visits by the family doctor for sudden acute problems or for dying patients, there are after-hours clinics and telehealth services, and end-of-life care is provided by hospices. Nurses, community pharmacists, and other primary care providers may have prescribing authority and be able to diagnose, investigate, and treat some conditions.

Furthermore, a doctor might choose family medicine as a career, at least made partly because of the flexibility of working hours and job-sharing possibilities. Many general practitioners only work part-time, and this, combined with high appointment numbers and often a general practitioner workforce shortage, means that patients are increasingly experiencing difficulties in getting an appointment with any doctor, let alone getting to consistently see their own general practitioner.[10]

Continuity in primary care is increasingly being viewed as a team-based effort rather than solely the responsibility of individual providers. Even if a particular practitioner is unavailable, the team can still provide consistent, comprehensive, and coordinated care over time. Strong, long-term relationships between patients and the care team provide continuity.[11]

Digitalisation in primary care can be considered a double-edged sword. It includes the electronic health record, which can be accessed and updated by all authorised health providers, ensuring that all team members are informed about the patient's status and treatment plans, improving coordination and continuity of care and preventing both duplication and fragmentation of services. Patient-centredness can be enhanced through online portals, enabling patients to access their medical records and track their own health, leading to better engagement and self-management. Telehealth can increase access, providing remote diagnosis and treatment of patients through telecommunications technology.

Along with the benefits, there are downsides to digitisation. Not all patients have equal access to these technologies, leading to a digital divide that exacerbates health inequities. Although there are secure platforms for information exchange, there are security concerns about sensitive information and potential data breaches, and reliance on these technologies rends the health system vulnerable should they fail. Online built-in guidelines and algorithms, such as those used in clinical decision support systems, may provide clinical advice based on the latest guidelines. However, they may reduce complex chronic care management to a series of siloed, disease-focused, formulaic decisions, undermining the core value of caring for patients in the context of their specific needs, circumstances, and preferences. Of particular concern, the use of digital tools may reduce face-to-face interactions between patients and their family physicians, hence reducing quality of care.

RESEARCH AND REFLECTIVITY

Values also need to be considered in research. Research is important for legitimacy of and training in family medicine locally, but it is also a strong foundation of the development of global family medicine. Its focus is on improving primary care practices and patient outcomes by addressing a wide range of health issues that affect individuals and families across their lifespan.

The domain of family medicine research is huge. It includes:

1. The ecology of medical care, its focus on the environments of healthcare, and interactions among them.
2. Causation and important opportunities to discover how people lose and regain their health.
3. Knowing medicine in different ways, focusing on what things mean in the inner and outer realities of individuals and groups of individuals.
4. The nature of the work of family physicians, such as first-contact care for any type of problem, sticking with patients regardless of their diagnoses, incorporating context into decision-making, developing relevant

technologies, articulating useful theory, and measuring what happens in family medicine.

5. The standard research categories of basic, clinical, health services, health policy, and educational research.
6. Thinking of family medicine research as both a linear process of translation and a wheel of knowledge with iterative loops of discovery that come from within family medicine.[12]

Family medicine research is essential for advancing primary care and ensuring that healthcare systems can meet the diverse needs of patients and communities. Billions of people will benefit from family medicine research.[12] Family medicine and primary care research is eclectic in its methodological approaches. Quantitative methods deal with numbers and may be used to measure health outcomes, prevalence of conditions, and the effectiveness of interventions. This research is considered to be objective. In qualitative methods the data are words and stories and are seen to be more subjective in nature. Qualitative methods are used to explore patient experiences, to understand healthcare provider perspectives, and to investigate the context of healthcare delivery.

Family medicine researchers were early adopters of mixed methods, with the systematic integration of quantitative and qualitative findings, as a distinct research approach.[13] The importance of combining both numbers and narratives to capture the nuanced and multi-faceted nature of primary care was recognized as important to address the complexities of family medicine.[14]

The influence of the researcher on the research process is well accepted in qualitative research. A positionality statement is common – acknowledging how the researchers' social and political context, including ethnicity, gender, and personal experiences, might have shaped their worldview and, consequently, the research process and outcomes. Reflexivity goes beyond this, making that positionality explicit. It is an ongoing critical thinking process, being aware of and questioning how the researchers' beliefs and values might be shaping their research decisions and interpretations, reflecting on the influence their positionality, biases, and interactions with participants might have on the findings.

As discussed earlier, values are always embedded in research. Even meta-analyses are not value-free.[15] Reflexivity should also take place in the more objective quantitative research, as well as in more subjective narrative-based qualitative studies. This will help address potential biases. Such transparency will enhance the credibility and ethical rigour of a study.

Increasingly, attention has been given to research that is directly applicable and relevant to people in the community in the context of their lives. Co-design approaches involve stakeholders such as community members, patients, and primary care providers as equal research partners, who generate the research questions and assist in answering them.[16,17] Community engagement ensures that interventions are culturally appropriate and address the specific needs of the population. Patient-centred approaches prioritize patients' needs and values and develop interventions tailored to their specific contexts. In parallel to clinical developments, there is a progressive move towards interdisciplinary and transdisciplinary collaboration of family medicine researchers with those from many other primary health and social care backgrounds in the team, who all bring their own perspectives, values, and biases to the table.

WONCA's International Classification System for Primary Care (ICPC) enables family physicians to code the reason for an encounter, episodes of care, symptoms, complaints, diagnosis, treatment, and other aspects of consultations. For countries that use this system, ICPC provides a rich dataset, granting knowledge of a patient's journey through the health system, sometimes over many years. This is a research resource that can also be used in combination or linkage with other datasets such as national registers. Coding using ICPC can render visibility of the core values of the family medicine profession by enabling consistent monitoring of the course of disease development and of continuity of care in personal relationship settings.

Reflectivity is just as important for knowledge transfer, when an intervention is to be implemented, to look at the meaning and implications of the research, its applicability, and its relevance to people in the context of their lives. Continuous evaluation and feedback loops with critical assessment of processes and outcomes can help refine interventions and address patients' needs and will ensure they remain relevant and effective over time.

In some countries there has been a growing divide between the academic units of family medicine at the universities and clinical practice at the grassroots. It is important that the research questions being addressed by these units are relevant and applicable to the communities they serve and are grounded in the principles of generalism, not a biomedical, disease-oriented approach.

FINDING COMMONALITY AMONG THE DIFFERENCES

The differences in peoples, their cultures, and values across the world are reflected in the core values and principles in family medicine determined in our regional chapters. There is considerable diversity in practice and in training within and across the regions in our discipline.

However, we can be enriched rather than hampered by our differences. Within this heterogeneity, we need a common identity for the recognition of our specialty and for advocacy, a common language of our humanity enabling us to connect with our colleagues across the world. Family medicine is a discipline but sometimes it is also a social movement, for example, advocating for improving equity of care and resources.[8]

IN CONCLUSION

Family medicine/primary care is the means to achieve universal health coverage, the goal of the World Health Organization (WHO).[18] However, globalization means that societal changes hit us all at a great pace and impact differently on our cultures, on our health systems, and on the ways we can live our lives. Healthcare, and first of all primary care, is always influenced and affected by societal trends.

Family medicine is a medical speciality, but it also needs to be a social movement to be able to counter undesirable trends that impact on the provision of healthcare for all.[8] To achieve this, family doctors need to have a clear understanding of the global common denominator of our discipline. This book is a step along the way to inspire continuing brainstorming and reflections on the foundation of family medicine and how it can be adapted and implemented in local contexts. Strong primary healthcare is important for society and for global stability.

REFERENCES

1. Greenhalgh T. Commentary: Without values, complexity is reduced to mathematics. *J Eval Clin Pract* 2025;31(1):e14263. https://doi.org/10.1111/jep.14263
2. Fulford K. Ten principles of values-based medicine. In: Radden J, ed. The Philosophy of Psychiatry: A Companion. New York: Oxford University Press 2004.
3. Fulford K, Peile E, Caroll H. Essential Values-Based Practice. Cambridge: Cambridge University Press 2021.
4. Hurst L, Mahtani K, Pluddemann A, et al. Defining Value-based Healthcare in the NHS: Centre for Evidence-Based Medicine Report. University of Oxford 2019.
5. Mohanna K. Values based practice: A framework for thinking with. *Educ Prim Care* 2017;28(4):192–6. https://doi.org/10.1080/14739879.2017.1313689
6. Stange KC, Ferrer RL. The paradox of primary care. *Ann Fam Med* 2009;7(4):293–9. https://doi.org/10.1370/afm.1023
7. Etz R, Miller WL, Stange KC. Simple rules that guide generalist and specialist care. *Fam Med* 2021;53(8):697–700. https://doi.org/10.22454/FamMed.2021.463594
8. Stange K. Generalism: What patients and clinicians say matters. WONCA Global Core Values Project. Zoom presentation, Dec 2024.
9. Starfield B. Primary Care: Balancing Health Needs, Services and Technology. New York, NY: Oxford University Press 1998.
10. Hutchinson J, Gibson J, Kontopantelis E, et al. Trends in full-time working in general practice: A repeated cross-sectional study. *Br J Gen Pract* 2024;74(747):e652. https://doi.org/10.3399/BJGP.2023.0432
11. Khatri R, Endalamaw A, Erku D, et al. Continuity and care coordination of primary health care: A scoping review. *BMC Health Serv Res* 2023;23(1):750. https://doi.org/10.1186/s12913-023-09718-8
12. Green LA. The research domain of family medicine. *Ann Fam Med* 2004;2(Suppl 2):S23. https://doi.org/10.1370/afm.147

13. Craddock Lee SJ. Mixed methods: Capturing complexity in family medicine research. *Ann Fam Med* 2021;19(2):98. https://doi.org/10.1370/afm.2682

14. Cresswell J. Research Design: Qualitative, Quantitative and Mixed Methods Approaches. 1st ed. Thousand Oaks, CA: Sage Publications 1994.

15. Goodyear-Smith FA, van Driel ML, Arroll B, et al. Analysis of decisions made in meta-analyses of depression screening and the risk of confirmation bias: A case study. *BMC Med Res Methodol* 2012;12. https://doi.org/10.1186/1471-2288-12-76

16. Lamont R, Fishman T, Sanders PF, et al. View from the canoe: Co-designing research pacific style. *Ann Fam Med* 2020;18(2):172–5. https://doi.org/10.1370/afm.2497

17. Tu'akoi S, Ofanoa M, Ofanoa S, et al. Co-designing an intervention to prevent rheumatic fever in pacific people in South Auckland: A study protocol. *Int J Equity Health* 2022;21(101):1–6. https://doi.org/10.1186/s12939-022-01701-9

18. World Health Organization Western Pacific Region. Universal Health Coverage: Moving towards Better Health Action Framework for the Western Pacific Region. Geneva: WHO, 2016:92.

WONCA member organizations by region

AFRICA

Botswana

Botswana Association of Family Physicians (BAOFP)

Cameroon

Medcamer Family Medicine (MFM)

Ghana

Society of Family Physicians of Ghana (SOFPOG)

Kenya

Kenya Association of Family Physicians (KAFP)

Lesotho

Lesotho Medical Association

Liberia

Society of Family Physicians of Liberia (SOFPOL)

Nigeria

Association of Nigerian Private Medical Practitioners (ANPMP)
National Postgraduate Medical College of Nigeria, Faculty of Family
    Medicine (NPMCN – FM)
Society of Family Physicians of Nigeria (SOFPON)

South Africa

South African Academy of Family Physicians (SAAFP)

Uganda

Association of Family Physicians of Uganda (AFPU)

Zambia

Association of Family Physicians of Zambia (AFPZ)

Zimbabwe

The College of Primary Care Physicians of Zimbabwe (CPCPZ)

ASIA PACIFIC

Australia

Australian College of Rural and Remote Medicine (ACRRM)
The Royal Australian College of General Practitioners (RACGP)

China

Chinese Medical Doctor Association General Practitioners Sub-Association (CMDA-GP)
Chinese Society of General Practice (CSGP)
General Practice Branch of Cross-Strait Medicine Exchange Association (SMEA-GP)

Fiji

Fiji College of General Practitioners (FCGP)

Hong Kong

The Hong Kong College of Family Physicians (HKCFP)

Indonesia

Indonesian Society of Teachers in Family Medicine (KIKLPI)
The Indonesian Association of Family Physicians (IAFP)

Japan

Japan Primary Care Association (JPCA)

Korea

The Korean Academy of Family Medicine (KAFM)

Macau

Macau Association of General Practitioners (AMCGM)

Malaysia

The Malaysian Family Medicine Specialists' Association (FMSA)
Academy of Family Physicians of Malaysia (AFPM)

Mongolia

Mongolian Association of Family Medicine Specialists (MAFMS)

Myanmar

Myanmar Medical Association, General Practitioners' Society (MMA-GPS)

New Zealand

The Royal New Zealand College of General Practitioners (RNZCGP)

Philippines

Philippine Academy of Family Physicians (PAFP)
Foundation For Family Medicine Educators, Inc (FAMed)

Singapore

College of Family Physicians Singapore (CFPS)

Taiwan

Chinese Taipei Association of Family Medicine (CTAFM)

Thailand

The General Practitioners/Family Physicians Association of Thailand (GPFPT)

Vietnam

Vietnam Association of Family Physicians (VAFP)

EAST MEDITERRANEAN

Afghanistan

Afghanistan Family Medicine Association (AFMA)

Algeria

Algerian Society of General Medicine (Société Algérienne de Médecine Générale) (ex-member)

Bahrain

Bahrain Family Physicians Association

Egypt

Egyptian Family Medicine Association (EFMA)

Iraq

Iraqi Family Physicians Society (IFPS)

Islamic Republic of Iran

Iranian Society of General Practitioner

Jordan

Jordan Society of Family Medicine (JSFM)

Kuwaiti

Kuwait Association of Family Physicians and General Practitioners (KSFGP)

Lebanon

Lebanese Society of Family Medicine (LSFM)

Morocco

National Collective of General Practitioners of Morocco (MG Maroc)

Oman

Oman Family and Community Medicine Society

Palestine

Palestinian Association of Family Medicine (PAFM)

Saudi Arabia

Saudi Society of Family and Community Medicine (SSFCM)

Syria

Syrian Association of Family Medicine

United Arab Emirates

Emirates Family Medicine Society (EFMS)

EUROPE

Armenia

Armenian Association of Family Physicians (ArmAFP)

Austria

Austrian Society of General Practice and Family Medicine (OEGAM)

Belgium

Belgian Society for General Practitioners (BSGP)

Bosnia & Herzegovina

Association of Family Physicians of the Federation of Bosnia & Herzegovina (UDP/OM)
Association of Family Physicians of Republic of Srpska

Bulgaria

Bulgarian General Practice Society for Research and Education (BGPSRE)

Croatia

Croatian Association of Family Medicine (HUOM)
Croatian Family Physicians Coordination (KoHOM)

Czech Republic

Czech Society of General Practice CLS JEP (CSGP)

Denmark

Danish College of General Practitioners (DSAM)

Estonia

Estonian Family Doctors Society (ESFD)

Finland

Finnish Association for General Practice (SYLY)

France

Collège de la Médecine Générale (CMG) French College of General Practice

Georgia

Georgia Family Medicine Association (GFMA)

Germany

German College of General Practitioners and Family Physicians (DEGAM)

Greece

Greek Association of General Practitioners (ELEGEIA)
Greek College of General Practitioners (GCGP)
Hippocrates, Association of General Practice/Family Medicine of Greece (EGOIE)

Hungary

Hungarian Research Organization of Family Physicians (CSAKOSZ)

Iceland

Icelandic College of Family Physicians (FIH)

Ireland

Irish College of General Practitioners (ICGP)

Israel

Israel Association of Family Physicians

Italy

Accademia Italiana Cure Primarie – ETS

Kazakhstan

Kazakhstan Association of Family Physicians (KAFP)

Kosovo

Association of Family Physicians of Kosovo (AFPK/AMFK)

Latvia

Rural Family Doctors Association of Latvia

Lithuania

Lithuanian College of Family Physicians (LSGK)

Luxembourg

Societé Scientifique Luxembourgeoise de Médecine Générale (SSLMG)

Malta

Malta College of Family Doctors (MCFD)

Netherlands

Dutch College of General Practitioners (DCGP/NHG)

North Macedonia

Association of Doctors of General Practitioners of Macedonia (ZLOM SM)

Norway

Norwegian College of General Practice (NFA)

Poland

The College of Family Physicians in Poland

Portugal

Portuguese Association of General Practice and Family Medicine (APMGF)

Tajikistan

Public Organization National Association of Family Medicine Workers of Tajikistan (NAFMST)

Romania

Romanian National Society of Family Medicine (SNMF)

Russia

All-Russian Fund – Association of General Practitioners of Russian Federation (RAGP)

Serbia

Section of General Practice of Serbian Medical Society

Slovakia

Slovak Society of General Practice (SkSGP/SSVPL)

Slovenia

The Slovenian Medical Association Slovenian Association of Family Physicians (ZZDM)

Spain

Sociedad Española de Médicos de Atención Primaria (SEMERGEN)
Spanish Society of Family and Community Medicine (SEMFYC)

Sweden

Swedish College of General Practice (SFAM)

Switzerland

Swiss Society of General Internal Medicine (SGAIM)

Türkiye

Turkish Association of Family Physicians (TAHUD)

Ukraine

Ukrainian Association of Family Medicine (UAFM)

United Kingdom

Royal College of General Practitioners (RCGP)

LATIN AMERICA

Argentina

Argentine Federation of Family and General Medicine (FAMFyG)

Bolivia

Bolivian Society of Family Medicine (SOBOMEFA)

Brazil

Brazilian Society of Family and Community Medicine (SBMFC)

Chile

Scientific Society of Family and General Medicine of Chile (SOCHIMEF)

Colombia

Colombian Society of Family Medicine (SOCMEF)

Costa Rica

Costa Rican Association of Specialists in Family and Community Medicine (MEDFAMCOMCR)

Cuba

Cuban Society of Family Medicine (SOCUMEFA)

Dominican Republic

Dominican Society of Family and Community Medicine (SODOMEFA)

Ecuador

Ecuador Society of Family Medicine (SEMF)

Mexico

Mexican Federation of Family Medicine Specialists and Residents (FMERMF)

Nicaragua

Nicaraguan Association of Family Medicine

Panama

Panamanian Association of Family Medicine

Paraguay

Paraguayan Society of Family Medicine (SPMF)

Peru

Peruvian Society of Family and Community Medicine (SOPEMFYC)

Uruguay

Uruguayan Society of Family Medicine (SUMEFAC)

Venezuela

Venezuelan Society of Family Medicine (SOVEMEFA)

NORTH AMERICA

Canada

The College of Family Physicians of Canada (CFPC)
Section of Teachers & Section of Researchers (STSR)

Jamaica (with chapters in Trinidad and Tobago, Barbados, and Bahamas)

The Caribbean College of Family Physicians (CCFP)

United States

American Academy of Family Physicians (AAFP)
American Board of Family Medicine (ABFM)

Association of Departments of Family Medicine (ADFM)
Society of Teachers of Family Medicine (STFM)

SOUTH ASIA
Bangladesh

Bangladesh College of General Practitioners (BCGP)

India

Academy of Family Physicians of India (AFPI)
Indian Medical Association College of General Practitioners

Nepal

General Practice and Emergency Medicine Association of Nepal (GPAN)

Pakistan

Pakistan Society of Family Physicians, Lahore (PSFP)
College of Family Medicine Pakistan (CFMP)

Sri Lanka

College of General Practitioners of Sri Lanka (CGPSL)

Index

Note: page numbers in *italics* indicate figures and page numbers in **bold** indicate tables on the corresponding pages.